Gluteal Augmentation

Editors

ASHKAN GHAVAMI
PAT PAZMINO
NEIL M. VRANIS

CLINICS IN PLASTIC SURGERY

www.plasticsurgery.theclinics.com

October 2023 • Volume 50 • Number 4

ELSEVIER

1600 John F. Kennedy Boulevard • Suite 1800 • Philadelphia, Pennsylvania, 19103-2899

http://www.theclinics.com

CLINICS IN PLASTIC SURGERY Volume 50, Number 4
October 2023 ISSN 0094-1298, ISBN-13: 978-0-443-13063-2

Editor: Stacy Eastman
Developmental Editor: Anita Chamoli

Clinics in Plastic Surgery (ISSN 0094-1298) is published quarterly by Elsevier Inc., 360 Park Avenue South, New York, NY 10010-1710. Months of issue are January, April, July, and October. Business and Editorial Offices: 1600 John F. Kennedy Blvd., Suite 1800, Philadelphia, PA 19103-2899. Periodicals postage paid at New York, NY and additional mailing offices. Subscription prices are $559.00 per year for US individuals, $1024.00 per year for US institutions, $100.00 per year for US students and residents, $625.00 per year for Canadian individuals, $1218.00 per year for Canadian institutions, $696.00 per year for international individuals, $1218.00 per year for international institutions, $100.00 per year for Canadian Students and $305.00 per year for international students/residents. To receive student/resident rate, orders must be accompanied by name of affiliated institution, date of term, and the *signature* of program/residency coordinator on institution letterhead. Orders will be billed at individual rate until proof of status is received. Foreign air speed delivery is included in all *Clinics* subscription prices. All prices are subject to change without notice. **POSTMASTER:** Send address changes to *Clinics in Plastic Surgery*, Elsevier Health Sciences Division, Subscription Customer Service, 3251 Riverport Lane, Maryland Heights, MO 63043. **Customer Service: 1-800-654-2452 (US and Canada). From outside of the United States and Canada, call 314-447-8871. Fax: 314-447-8029. E-mail: JournalsCustomerService-usa@elsevier.com (for print support); JournalsOnlineSupport-usa@elsevier.com (for online support).**

Reprints. For copies of 100 or more of articles in this publication, please contact the Commercial Reprints Department, Elsevier Inc., 360 Park Avenue South, New York, New York 10010-1710. Tel.: +1-212-633-3874; Fax: +1-212-633-3820; E-mail: reprints@elsevier.com.

Clinics in Plastic Surgery is covered in *Current Contents, EMBASE/Excerpta Medica, Science Citation Index, MEDLINE/PubMed (Index Medicus), ASCA,* and *ISI/BIOMED.*

Contributors

EDITORS

ASHKAN GHAVAMI, MD
Assistant Clinical Professor, Department of
Surgery, Division of Plastic and Reconstructive
Surgery, David Geffen School of Medicine at
UCLA, Los Angeles, California, USA; Private
Practice, Ghavami Plastic Surgery, Beverly
Hills, California, USA

PAT PAZMINO, MD
Department of Surgery, Division of Plastic and
Reconstructive Surgery, University of Miami,
Miller School of Medicine, Private Practice,
Miami Aesthetic, Miami, Florida, USA

NEIL M. VRANIS, MD
Private Practice, Ghavami Plastic Surgery,
Beverly Hills, California, USA

AUTHORS

ALEXANDER ASLANI, MD, PhD
Director, Cirumed Clinic Marbella, Marbella,
Málaga, Spain

HÉCTOR CÉSAR DURÁN VEGA, MD
Plastic Surgeon in Private Practice, ASAPS,
ASPS, AMCPER, FILACP, Centro Medico de
Las Americas CMA, Merida, Yucatán, Mexico

STEFAN DANILLA, MD, MSc
Cirujano Plástico Magíster en Epidemiología
Clínica, Clínica AUREA, Santiago, Chile

DANIEL DEL VECCHIO, MD, MBA
Attending Surgeon, Department of Plastic
Surgery, Massachusetts General Hospital,
Boston, Massachusetts, USA

ASHKAN GHAVAMI, MD
Assistant Clinical Professor, Department of
Surgery, Division of Plastic and Reconstructive
Surgery, David Geffen School of Medicine at
UCLA, Los Angeles, California; Private
Practice, Ghavami Plastic Surgery, Beverly
Hills, California, USA

ALFREDO E. HOYOS ARIZA, MD
Plastic Surgeon, CEO at Total Definer Medical,
Member of the Colombian Society of Plastic,
Aesthetic, Maxillofacial, and Hand Surgery,
Member of the American Society of Plastic

Surgeons (ASPS), Private Practice, Bogota,
Colombia

DIANA MICHELI, MD
Equipo de Cirugia Plástica, Pontificia
Universidad Catolica, Santiago, Chile

PAT PAZMIÑO, MD
Department of Surgery, Division of Plastic and
Reconstructive Surgery, University of Miami,
Miller School of Medicine, Private Practice,
Miami Aesthetic, Miami, Florida, USA

MAURICIO PEREZ PACHON, MD
Doctor and Surgeon, Head, Scientific
Department at Total Definer Medical, Bogota,
Colombia; Mayo Clinic, Department of
Surgery, Rochester, Minnesota, USA

DOUGLAS STEINBRECH, MD
New York Institute of Male Plastic Surgery,
New York, New York, USA

DAVID M. STEPIEN, MD, PhD
Assistant Professor, Division of Plastic,
Maxillofacial, and Oral Surgery, Duke
University

NEIL M. VRANIS, MD
Private Practice, Ghavami Plastic Surgery,
Beverly Hills, California, USA

Contents

> Gluteal fat grafting is the fastest growing surgery in body contouring because of the powerful results that no other procedure can achieve. Efforts made to improve the safety of this procedure are reviewed.

> Demand for autologous gluteal augmentation with fat transfer continues to rise paralleling the increasingly complex nature of the operation. Improved overall aesthetic outcomes are a result of: (1) donor site fat harvest has evolved to circumferential torso high-definition lipo-sculpting; (2) a shift from indiscriminate buttock augmentation to precise gluteal re-shaping. Discussing complex operations with patients, particularly ones of artistic nature, can be challenging. The senior author has developed a gluteal re-shaping graphic to focus a patient's attention to the four most important areas. It also serves as a foundation for surgeons to create operative plans and track outcomes for professional development.

> This article explores the importance of understanding the tridimensional artistic anatomy of the back, pelvis, and thighs in gluteal surgery. It emphasizes the need for plastic surgeons to have a comprehensive knowledge of these anatomic structures to achieve successful outcomes. The authors highlight the significance of ethnic differences in determining ideal aesthetic results and stress the importance of considering and respecting these variations. Individualization of treatment is a key principle in gluteal surgery, as each patient has unique preferences and needs. Effective communication and collaboration between the surgeon and the patient are crucial in determining desired aesthetic goals and achieving satisfactory outcomes.

> Gluteal contouring has been subject to numerous publications in aesthetic plastic surgery. Not only the female but also the male features that govern such procedures have been thoroughly described by different authors. In this article, we will provide the reader with an updated account of how gluteal contouring blends with High Definition Liposculpture (HDL). We discuss the most current techniques for buttocks reshaping through a holistic approach of new anatomical and artistic concepts. We will dive into new techniques to perform multiplanar and 4-dimensional Fat Grafting and equalization of the buttocks and surrounding areas, which we believe might help

plastic surgeons to improve the quality of their patient outcomes. In effect, a proper understanding of the anatomical structures and its variations among different gender and ethnicities, will both help the surgeon to individualize the procedure based on patient preferences.

Liposuction cannulas are versatile tools in a plastic surgeon's armamentarium useful for dissection, deep subcutaneous ligamentous release, fat extraction, and lipofilling. Experienced surgeons develop the ability to navigate subcutaneous anatomy through real-time tactile feedback of the cannula's depth, angulation, excursion, and resistance. Peripheral gluteal ligaments acting as anatomic boundaries must be understood and protected. However, central ligaments tether the dermis to deeper structures precluding expansion. Appropriate, targeted ligamentous weakening improves focal capacitance allowing precise gluteal contouring while staying in safe planes. This maneuver is critical during subcutaneous lipofilling of the S-Curve® procedure to create an aesthetically pleasing, convex gluteal silhouette.

 Video content accompanies this article at http://www.plasticsurgery.theclinics.com.

Guidelines for optimal buttock implant management, time-efficient preparation of implant pocket, and breakdown of optimal implant choice, combined with large-volume fat transfer for best possible outcome.

 Video content accompanies this article at http://www.plasticsurgery.theclinics.com.

The concept of the gluteal framework has significantly enhanced our understanding of the gluteal anatomy. The buttock does not constitute a bulging area in the human body. To be attractive, it must harmonize with all elements of the human body around it. Nevertheless, the changes in patient desires and demands, in addition to innovations in surgical technique open a field of opportunity to achieve more beautiful and natural results. In this work, the main updates in the management of body contouring are condensed, including new safe and aesthetic fat infiltration techniques.

Low-cost, high-resolution ultrasound systems allow surgeons to visualize and manipulate the subcutaneous space and inject fat graft with millimeter accuracy.

Static injection, migration, and equalization allows for always subcutaneous-targeted fat grafting to either the deep or the superficial subcutaneous spaces.

The shape and definition of the male buttock have been emphasized throughout time, as it represents masculinity, strength, health, and beauty across various cultures. Aesthetic Plastic Surgery in general has become more acceptable for men; thus, the demand for gluteal enhancement parallels this shift in social norms. Surgeons interested in such cases must first understand the aesthetic ideals and principles of gluteal shaping as it pertains to men. By using gluteal implants, fat transfer techniques, local tissue rearrangement principles, or a combination thereof, one can sculpt an aesthetically pleasing male buttock with a high degree of patient satisfaction.

Gluteal augmentation is a quickly evolving field that continues to grow in the realms of patient safety, surgical education, and technological advancement. This article discusses innovation in gluteal augmentation and suggests potential new pathways for developing the practice of gluteal augmentation.

CLINICS IN PLASTIC SURGERY

Preface
Gluteal Augmentation: Optimizing Safety and Aesthetics

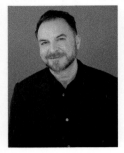
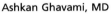
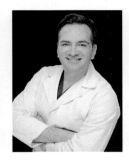
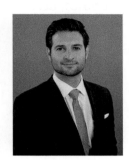

Ashkan Ghavami, MD   Pat Pazmino, MD   Neil M. Vranis, MD

Editors

Gluteal augmentation has become an increasingly popular operation with the unfortunate stigmata that it carries unacceptably high morbidity and mortality rates. Basic gluteal augmentation procedures with the sole purpose of increasing size, and in particular projection, by indiscriminately adding large volumes of fat (and/or implants) are a trend of the past. These procedures have since evolved. They have become more sophisticated and nuanced. By understanding anatomic boundaries and respecting internal structures, a well-trained, meticulous surgeon can consistently deliver aesthetically pleasing results. This philosophy also promotes longevity of the operated buttock. Elegant and harmonious contours of the torso and gluteal region can be achieved using implants, fat transfer, or a combination thereof. Performing these procedures properly can significantly mitigate the risks and associated downstream sequelae. Establishing appropriate safeguards and teaching proper technique are of utmost importance for enhancing gluteal aesthetics with high patient satisfaction.

Social media, heightened patient expectations, and the desire for excellence have challenged surgeons performing these operations to push the frontier to achieve more natural and finessed results. Liposuction performed as an ancillary procedure or for the purpose of fat harvest is of equal importance to establish desirable waist-to-hip ratios and athletic abdominal contouring that complement the newly created buttock size and shape.

This issue focuses on maximizing safety and how to implement the most current and innovative techniques for gluteal augmentation. Surgeons interested in safely pushing the boundaries while optimizing outcomes will greatly benefit as they extract nuanced pearls from masters in this field. Topics covered include safety, preoperative considerations/ideal aesthetics, regional liposculpting, total body contouring, combining implants with fat transfer, the role of technology (ie, ultrasound, skin-tightening devices, laser/ultrasound-assisted liposuction), male-specific considerations, and the challenge of managing complications associated with buttock augmentation.

We would like to thank all the contributors who have made it possible to create such a valuable resource, relevant to both the novice and the experienced surgeon who perform gluteal augmentation and body-contouring procedures.

Ashkan Ghavami, MD
Department of Surgery
Division of Plastic and Reconstructive Surgery
David Geffen School of Medicine at UCLA
Los Angeles, CA, USA

Ghavami Plastic Surgery
433 North Camden Drive, Suite 780
Beverly Hills, CA 90210, USA

Clin Plastic Surg 50 (2023) ix–x
https://doi.org/10.1016/j.cps.2023.07.006
0094-1298/23/© 2023 Published by Elsevier Inc.

plasticsurgery.theclinics.com

Pat Pazmino, MD
Department of Surgery
Division of Plastic and Reconstructive Surgery
University of Miami, Miller School of Medicine
Miami, FL, USA

Miami Aesthetic
848 Brickell Avenue, Suite 820
Miami, FL 33131, USA

Neil M. Vranis, MD
Ghavami Plastic Surgery
433 North Camden Drive, Suite 780
Beverly Hills, CA 90210, USA

E-mail addresses:
ashghavami@yahoo.com (A. Ghavami)
dr@miamia.com (P. Pazmino)
drvranis@gmail.com (N.M. Vranis)

Safety in Gluteal Augmentation

Pat Pazmiño, MD[a],*, Daniel Del Vecchio, MD, MBA[b,1]

KEYWORDS

- Brazilian butt lift • BBL • Gluteal fat grafting • Buttock augmentation • Buttock enlargement
- Safe Buttock Lipoaugmentation • Fat transfer • Ultrasound

KEY POINTS

- Gluteal fat grafting remains the fastest growing procedure in body contouring which allows for focal correction of asymmetried and global buttock enhancement.
- Gluteal fat grafting has had unusually high complication and mortality rates when surgeons inadvertently injected fat graft into the muscles and intramuscular veins.
- Cadaver studies, morgue autopsies, plastic surgery societies, and regulatory agencies have noted that fat graft should only be injected into the subcutaneous space above the deep gluteal fascia.
- Imaging technologies have been introduced to allow surgeons to confirm subcutaneous only fat graft placement.
- Florida became the first state to enact a law mandating that all gluteal fat grafting must be performed using ultrasound guidance.

Over the past 6 years, gluteal fat grafting, commonly referred to as a Brazilian Butt Lift or "BBL," has become one of the most popular and controversial procedures in esthetic surgery.[1,2] Although it can produce dramatic results, the consequences are sometimes fatal if not done correctly. Due to this, the BBL has been criticized in the media and even banned by some plastic surgery organizations.[3–5]

In October 2018, the British Association of Aesthetic Plastic Surgeons recommended that their members stop performing BBLs because of the reported high mortality rate of this blind procedure.[6] UK patients traveled to Turkey, Spain, and other countries for their BBL procedures. The British experience demonstrated that when trained plastic surgeons avoid this procedure, patients seek care from surgeons in other countries with less oversight.[7]

Multiple plastic surgery societies (ASAPS, ASPS, ISAPS, ISPRES, and IFATS) published guidelines that emphasized that fat graft must only be injected above the muscle in the subcutaneous layer.[8] In 2019, the Florida Board of Medicine (FL BOM) mandated that all gluteal fat grafting be performed only in the subcutaneous space. The FL BOM revisited this issue in 2022 with an emergency order detailing how to technically perform this surgery and limiting the number of procedures a surgeon could perform in a day, creating the precedent for legislative limitations on medical procedures.[9]

The dilemma gluteal surgeons faced was that cadaver studies, morgue autopsies, society guidelines, and Board of Medicine orders mandated *where* the fat graft should be placed, but did not show surgeons *how* to accurately and consistently inject fat graft in the subcutaneous space. This lack of total certainty as to the safe and correct placement of fat graft was the final obstacle in making the BBL safe, efficient, accurate, consistent, and teachable.

Advances in ultrasound imaging technology have helped to fill this safety gap. Over the last 5 years, ultrasound probes have entered the market, which use inexpensive arrays of crystals or microchips

[a] Division of Plastic Surgery, University of Miami; [b] Department of Plastic Surgery, Massachusetts General Hospital, Boston, MA, USA
[1] Present address: 38 Newbury Street, Suite 502, Boston, MA 02116.
* Corresponding author. 848 Brickell Avenue, Suite 820 Miami, FL 33131.
E-mail address: cps@miamia.com

Clin Plastic Surg 50 (2023) 521–523
https://doi.org/10.1016/j.cps.2023.07.001

Abbreviations	
ASAPS	The Aesthetic Society
APSPS	American Society of Plastic Surgery
ISAPS	International Society of Aesthetic Plastic Surgery
ISPRES	International Society of Plastic Regenerative Surgeons
IFATS	International Federation for Adipose Therapeutics and Science

to generate ultrasound waves and have coupled this technology with artificial intelligence to optimize image clarity and wireless connectivity to control the device from a smartphone or tablet. These devices can be readily used in the clinic or the sterile environment of the operating room. For the first time, affordable portable ultrasound probes allowed surgeons to visualize their fat grafting cannula and ensure that fat is placed subcutaneously in every patient, every time. The ease of use of portable ultrasound and its rapid adoption motivated the British Association of Aesthetic Plastic Surgeons to reverse their ban on BBLs and encouraged their member surgeons to only perform gluteal fat grafting with ultrasound guidance.[10]

In 2022, the FL BOM noted this novel safety feature when they issued an emergency order stating that all gluteal fat grafting must be performed with ultrasound guidance.[11] Ultrasound-guided gluteal fat grafting quickly became the standard of care in Florida. This was affirmed on June 28, 2023, when Florida Governor DeSantis signed into law House Bill 1471 that mandated the use of ultrasound with every gluteal fat grafting procedure.[12] The rapid adoption of ultrasound technology into this previously blind surgical procedure underscored the deep concern and high interest of both surgeons and legislators to make this popular procedure safe and consistent. Ultrasound can not only make gluteal surgeons safer but also by allowing them to visualize and manipulate gluteal anatomy, better surgeons.[13]

CLINICS CARE POINTS

- When performing gluteal fat grafting, consider the subcutaneous anatomy and understand the target zone for subcutaneous fat grafting.
- Create a treatment plan to confirm consistent subcutaneous placement of fat graft.

DISCLOSURE

The authors have nothing to disclose. Consultant: Clarius Mobile Health.

REFERENCES

1. The Aesthetic Society. Aesthetic plastic surgery national databank 2021. Aesthetic Surg J 2022; 42(Supp 1):1–18. Accessed October 10, 2022. https://cdn.theaestheticsociety.org/media/statistics/2021-TheAestheticSocietyStatistics.pdf.
2. Ghavami A, Villanueva NL. Gluteal augmentation and contouring with autologous fat transfer: part I. Clin Plast Surg 2018;45(2):249–59.
3. Dubrow T. "Botched" Star Terry Dubrow Warns Brazilian Butt Lift Could Kill You. TMZ. Published 2021. Available at: https://www.tmz.com/2021/05/31/botched-dr-terry-dubrow-warning-brazilian-butt-lift-kill-you-most-dangerous-operation/. Accessed July 24, 2022.
4. Saltz R. "Patient Alert: Gluteal Fat Grafting To The Buttocks Is A. Premier Physician Marketing. Published 2018. Available at: https://www.globenewswire.com/news-release/2018/08/30/1563640/0/en/Patient-Alert-Gluteal-Fat-Grafting-To-The-Buttocks-Is-A-High-Risk-Cosmetic-Surgery-Procedure-Warns-International-Society-of-Aesthetic-Plastic-Surgery-ISAPS.html. Accessed September 4, 2022.
5. Brucculieri J. Brazilian Butt Lifts Are Resulting In An Alarmingly High Mortality Rate | HuffPost Life. Huffington Post. Published 2018. Available at: https://www.huffpost.com/entry/brazilian-butt-lift-risks_n_5b6c39c1e4b0530743c77cf6. Accessed July 24, 2022.
6. Chalmers V. Brazilian butt-lift surgeons warned fat must ONLY be injected under the skin or the procedure | Daily Mail Online. Daily Mail. Published 2019. Available at: https://www.dailymail.co.uk/health/article-7041193/Brazilian-butt-lift-surgeons-warned-fat-injected-skin-procedure.html. Accessed July 24, 2022
7. Tillo O, Nassab R, Pacifico MD. The british association of aesthetic plastic surgeons (BAAPS) Gluteal fat grafting safety review and recommendations. Aesthetic Surg J 2022. https://doi.org/10.1093/ASJ/SJAC316.
8. Mills D, Rubin P, Saltz R. Fat Grafting to the Buttocks | American Society of Plastic Surgeons. ASPS. Published 2018. Available at: https://www.plasticsurgery.org/for-medical-professionals/advocacy/key-issues/fat-grafting-to-the-buttocks. Accessed July 24, 2022.
9. Florida Board of Medicine. 22065771, 64B8ER19-1 - Florida Administrative Rules, Law, Code, Register - FAC, FAR, eRulemaking. Florida Administrative Code & Florida Administrative Register. Published

2019. Available at: https://www.flrules.org/Gateway/View_notice.asp?id=22065771. Accessed September 4, 2022.

10. Tillo O, Nassab R, Pacifico MD. The British association of aesthetic plastic surgeons (BAAPS) gluteal fat grafting safety review and recommendations. Aesthetic Surg J 2023;43(6):675–82.

11. Florida Board of Medicine. 2022.06.08 64B8ER22-3 Florida Board of Medicine Emergency Rule on BBL. Florida Registrar. Published June 8, 2022. Available at: https://flboardofmedicine.gov/pdfs/64B8ER22-3-emergency-rule.pdf. Accessed June 28, 2023.

12. DeSantis R. Governor DeSantis Signs HB 1471. Florida Governors Office. Published June 28, 2022. Available at: https://www.flgov.com/2023/06/28/governor-desantis-signs-eight-bills-and-vetoes-one-bill/. Accessed June 28, 2023

13. Pazmiño P, Del Vecchio D. Static injection, migration, and equalization (SIME): a new paradigm for safe ultrasound-guided Brazilian butt lift: safer, faster, better. Aesthetic Surg J 2023. https://doi.org/10.1093/ASJ/SJAD142.

Patient Pre-operative Planning of Gluteal Augmentation

Ashkan Ghavami, MD[a,b,*], Neil M. Vranis, MD[b]

KEYWORDS

- Gluteal anatomy • S-Curve® • Pre-operative planning • Patient-surgeon communication
- Gluteal lipoaugmentation

KEY POINTS

- The pre-operative consultation for gluteal lipoaugmentation can be challenging to navigate given the highly artistic nature of the procedure.
- Simple and easy to understand illustrations enhance patient understanding of the procedure, align patient-surgeon expectations and help determine fat transfer prioritization when donor site adiposity is limited.
- Systematic reviews have demonstrated that patients benefit from concise yet precise informational leaflets to augment oral information provided by the surgeon.
- The Ghavami Gluteal Graphic was designed to help surgeons communicate with patients and to enhance patient understanding specifically for gluteal lipoaugmentation procedures.
- The graphic also allows surgeons to critically analyze surgical results and track the fidelity of anticipated surgical plan with actual operative execution in order to improve and refine techniques.

INTRODUCTION

In the early 2000's, gluteal augmentation gained significant attention in the media which has translated to a steady increase in surgical demand. The barometer for achieving excellent results, enhanced yet natural appearing contours, in gluteal lipo-augmentation cases has also risen. Performing liposuction for debulking or solely for the purpose of fat harvest has morphed into a sophisticated sculpting procedure. When performed well, areas of the body that hace been carefully lipo-sculpted complement the augmentation portion of the operation by highlighting the underlying musculature, bony edges, and their associated transitions. Similarly, gluteal augmentation began as a naive volume-enhancing procedure with the goal of adding fat throughout the entire buttocks, concentrating on achieving high rates of graft survival. Over time, these procedures have become more refined with an emphasis on precise, focal enhancements to create a well-balanced width-to-projection ratio that also complements the remainder of the patient's body (ie, waist and thighs). Advancing the frontiers for both portions of the procedure (liposuction and lipofilling) heightens the complexity of the operation and challenges the surgeon. Fortunately, surgical technique, appreciation for regional anatomy, and fat grafting principles continue to evolve leading to better-quality outcomes. This text reviews the importance of patient education and careful pre-operative analysis, especially how certain external contours correlate to predictable and consistent underlying anatomy.

[a] Department of Surgery, Division of Plastic and Reconstructive Surgery, David Geffen School of Medicine at UCLA, Los Angeles, CA, USA; [b] Private Practice, Ghavami Plastic Surgery, 433 North Camden Drive, Suite 780, Beverly Hills, CA 90210, USA
* Corresponding author. Department of Surgery, Division of Plastic and Reconstructive Surgery, David Geffen School of Medicine at UCLA, Los Angeles, CA.
E-mail address: ashghavami@yahoo.com

Clin Plastic Surg 50 (2023) 525–532
https://doi.org/10.1016/j.cps.2023.06.006
0094-1298/23/© 2023 Elsevier Inc. All rights reserved.

Succinct and effective patient communication during the consultation optimizes efficiency in the office while maintaining high patient satisfaction. It is customary for plastic surgeons to communicate anticipated results to patients through the use of visual simulations. This is very common before rhinoplasty and breast procedures through the use of photo editing software to generate renditions or the surgeon performs real-time artistic drawings of the patient's current anatomy versus the shape that they should expect after surgery. These maneuvers are an effort to ensure the alignment of patient expectations with the surgeon's vision. Particularly in the era where social media dominates, patients are constantly viewing images, illustrations, and photographs of themselves and others. Finding ways to incorporate visual aids into the consultation further buttresses the patient-surgeon relationship.

BACKGROUND

Patients present with various baseline gluteal shapes and sizes, influenced by their ethnicity, genetics, age, weight fluctuations and muscle tone. Age and weight gain increase the tendency to preferentially accumulate adiposity in the inferior pole of the buttock.[1] Standardizing descriptions of gluteal shape was initially attempted in 2006 when Mendieta[2] introduced the first classification system. It considers the patient's bony framework, size of gluteus maximus muscle, adipose topography, and skin quality. The gluteal shape is determined based on the relationship of the upper lateral hip width compared to the lateral leg width. The extrapolated line between these 2 points resembles the letters A or V and the width of the buttock at the midpoint determines if the shape is considered round or square relative to that imaginary line.[2] A limitation is that this classification system does not account for the other essential variable: size. Particularly, the size of the buttock relative to the waist. Width in the posterior view and projection on the lateral view play a significant role in the overall aesthetics even if the shape is optimized. Over the subsequent decade, various other authors have been published multiple iterations of a subunit principle applied to the buttock.[3–5] The most detailed one deliniated ten subunits including the back, buttock, and upper thigh.[5] It highlights the importance of considering the buttock in addition to adjacent regions ranging from the upper back to thighs when discussing posterior aesthetics.

The surgeon's ability to visualize underlying osseo-ligamentous anatomy and foresee their predictable effect translated to external contours is critical when performing gluteal contouring procedures. Bony landmarks such as the posterior superior iliac spine, iliac crest, and ischial tuberosity, have been used to reliably predict the superior and inferior borders of the buttock respectively.[1] Each buttocks is more than a simple, round, hemi-spherical structure. Shadows created by the depressions of the sacral triangle, sacral dimples, lateral trochanteric depression, midline gluteal cleft, and the medial infragluteal fold represent normal anatomy framing the borders of the buttock. Ghavami and colleagues performed a cadaveric study to identify and analyze the consistency of the main gluteal subcutaneous ligaments and adhesions that contribute to the internal structure and form the boundaries of each buttock. Their anatomic dissections consistently located four stout structures in the subcutaneous space: the sacrocutaneous ligament, the ischiocutaneous ligament, the gluteal cleft adhesion, and the inferior gluteal crease adhesion.[6]

The concept of anatomic subunits and fat compartments is well accepted for other parts of the body, in particular, the face. After Ghavami and colleagues described the presence and importance of gluteal ligaments,[6] additional cadaveric studies by other authors have been repeated.[3] Collectively, the various compartments contribute to the overall buttock shape and explain certain deformities when particular areas are inadvertently overfilled while adjacent areas are neglected. For example, the 'tombstone deformity' can occur when excess fat is preferentially transferred to the superolateral buttock without the adequate release of the mid-lateral depression/hollow.[7]

THE GHAVAMI GLUTEAL GRAPHIC

The gluteal graphic developed by the senior author was designed to be a simple yet effective communication tool useful for both the surgeon and patient. Gentle 'S'-shaped curves are observed in AP, PA, profile, and oblique views. When visualized from posterior, the 'S'-shape outline is formed from the concave curve of the back that gently merges with the convexity of the buttock. A natural yet attractive waist-to-hip width as seen from the posterior view ideally approximates the golden ratio of 1:1.6. Certain cultures appreciate slightly wider hips with ratios approaching 1:1.7. These minor differences are a matter of aesthetic taste and preference as long as the goal is to remain within a standard deviation of what is considered "normal" appearance. Key landmarks integrated into the diagram for reference include the sacrum, posterior iliac crest, and trochanteric depression (**Fig. 1**).

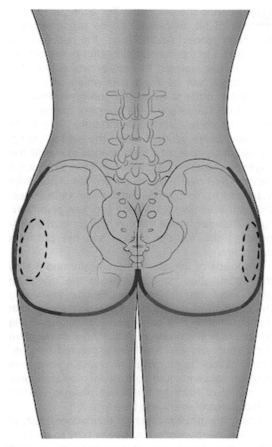

Fig. 1. An illustration of the posterior torso, buttocks and upper thighs showing the "ideal" surface contours in relation to the underlying pelvic bony anatomy. Also shown are the important bony and surface landmarks include the sacrum, posterior iliac crest, and trochanteric depression (*dotted ovals*).

Patients are often overwhelmed with information particularly when discussing operations that involve a large surface area or multiple body parts. To enhance patient comprehension, the senior author recommends focusing their attention specifically at the buttock and the immediate surrounding as this is their primary motivation for the consultation. Liposuction donor areas are of secondary concern and thus reviewed separately or even at a subsequent pre-operative visit.

The buttocks and thighs can be divided into 4 sections on each side (**Fig. 2**). Subdividing this region allows the patient and surgeon to focus their attention on particular areas of deficiency. This systematic method of analysis also highlights which areas require additional volume for optimal re-shaping. Territory 'A' resembles an upside down "L," covering the superior and medial areas

of the buttock. This is perhaps the most important area as it defines the lower back sacral "V," sets the height of the buttock and extends medially toward the center where projection is greatest. 'A' ' (A-prime) is an adjacent triangular subsection in the inferio-central and inferio-medial area that includes a notable zone of adhesion. This area is often challenging to expand in patients with stout ischiocutaneous ligaments. Territory 'B' represents the superio-lateral quadrant with variable extension to the anterior thigh. It includes the transition from the narrowest point of the flank to the point of maximal convexity at the gluteal mid-lateral point. Mendieta refers to this point as 'Point C' when he originally classified the various buttock phenotypes that exist in the population.[2] Lastly, Territory 'C' includes the inferolateral quadrant. This denotes the lateral transition from buttock to upper thigh, an area often neglected in standard gluteal lipo-augmentation procedures. Similar to a Venn diagram, the three main territories coalesce at the center of the buttock which corresponds to the area of maximal projection. This peak of maximal projection should reside halfway between the inferior gluteal crease and upper gluteal edge.[8]

The diagram was designed to highlight the premise that the S-Curve® procedure does not only focus on the buttock, instead considers reshaping the buttock and adjacent areas from the upper back to the level of the mid-thigh. The two views (AP, PA) of the graphic have been used to customize the operative plan for each particular patient. Surgeons can use various colors to indicate areas that require debulking or expansion along with various symbols to represent specific anatomic observations (ie, pelvic tilt, innate volume differences) or zones that will require a more extensive ligamentous release (**Fig. 3**).

CLINICAL APPLICATION: THE GHAVAMI GLUTEAL GRAPHIC

For surgeons, the utility of the Ghavami Gluteal Graphic extends beyond the pre-operative consultation. During the operation it serves as a guide, reminding surgeons of observed anatomic asymmetries, zones of anticipated adherence, and areas of preferential lipofilling. In the post-operative setting, surgeons can utilize it as a tool to assess the fidelity between anticipated surgical plans, operative execution and long-term results.

Like any surgery, in order to establish a strong patient-surgeon relationship it is critical to set expectations and limitations of the procedure. This will typically occur during the pre-operative conversation. As procedural complexity increases with the addition of multiple variables and artistic

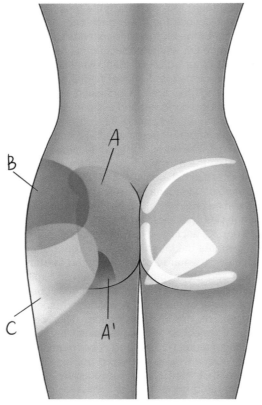

Fig. 2. The Ghavami Gluteal Graphic is an illustration of the posterior torso, buttock and upper thighs. The buttocks and associated transition points have been subdivided into four areas (A, B, C, A′). These are designed to help patients understand exactly which parts of their buttocks need to be augmented or reduced. The right buttock demonstrates the location of the most important gluteal ligaments and adhesions (the sacrocutaneous ligament, the ischiocutaneous ligament, the gluteal cleft adhesion, and the inferior gluteal crease adhesion).

creativity, it becomes even more important to develop efficient methods of communication to highlight pertinent details with patients, family members, media, and other non-medical professionals. The consultation must also emphasize and educate patients that the primary goal is re-shaping the buttock and nearby regions by carefully adding volume, width and projection to specific areas of deficiency rather than simply making the entire buttock bigger.[9] In order to achieve this, the diagram/graphic serves as an excellent visual aid to supplement verbal communication ensuring that the patient's desires and understanding align with the surgeon's vision.

The four subunits also permit the patient and surgeon to prioritize particular areas over others (**Fig. 4**). This is particularly useful in patients with

limited donor site adiposity. For example, a percentage of fat allocation can be predetermined for each zone. Additionally, the educational component of the consultation affords the opportunity to the surgeon to convey which areas of the buttock will be filled and which should be avoided in order to avoid disfigurement. Patients often do not understand the complex interplay between anatomy, addition/subtraction capability and how these variable affect the overall gluteal shape. Many present with demands to overfill the superior aspect of the buttock. F ailure to educate patients that overfilling the superolateral quadrant may lead to 'tombstone' and 'boxy' deformities. This pre-operative illustration tool can also highlight instances where there is high (or low) fidelity between the surgeon's plan and the patient's complaint.

Mark-ups of the diagram are performed during the consultation as one creates the operative plan. Inquisitive patients appreciate visualizing the creation of an operative blueprint along with the explanation that corresponds to diagramming which areas will undergo debulking with negative contouring and which will be expanded for optimum gluteal re-shaping. A pre-operative and post-operative marked up diagram may also serve as a way of tracking predictive planning versus actual surgical execution (see **Fig. 3**).

Lastly, the graphic has high educational utility in teaching inexperienced surgeons how to perform finessed gluteal augmentation procedures with autologous fat transfer. Previous schemes in the literature for marking patients involve too many landmarks that can be difficult to appreciate in obese patients or are too complex to remember/implement.[8] The simplicity of this method with four target zone can be easily transposed onto a patient's body (see **Fig. 4**). Creating a detailed topographic map highlighting regions that need excavation, expansion or internal release is useful in the pre-operative and intra-operative setting (see **Fig. 3**).

DISCUSSION

One of the challenges associated with any pre-operative consultation includes effective communication between both parties to establish alignment in expectations and anticipated outcomes. This is particularly difficult in procedures such as gluteal augmentation with autologous fat transfer given the highly artistic nature of the operation. Studies have found that surgeons of all specialties tailor their consultation with patients based on perceived competence and interpersonal behaviors.[10] A systematic review of 86 studies in the

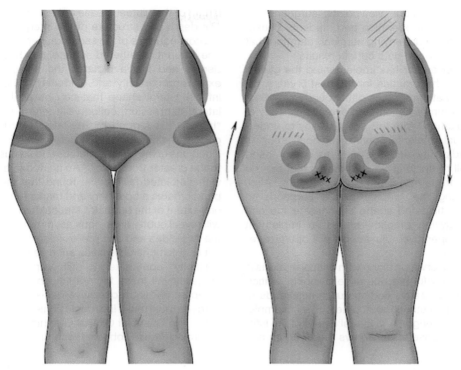

Fig. 3. An illustration that demonstrates the pre-operative planning/considerations in performing liposuction and gluteal augmentation via fat transfer. Red highlights the areas of reduction, while the green depicts which parts of the buttock will be infiltrated with fat. The arrows depict pelvic tilt and the 'xxx' are areas that will require extensive release due to strong osseocutaneous ligamentous attachment.

literature reported that the 3 essential factors patients use to select their surgeon are reputation, competency, and interpersonal skills.[11] This highlights the need for surgeons to cultivate excellent communication skills in addition to their surgical abilities. The use of illustrations and visual aids to supplement verbal communication during a consultation is not a novel concept. Standardized Gunter diagrams have been utilized in rhinoplasty for decades. Patients understand the anticipated

Scenario 1:

Priority	Surgeon	Patient
1	A / A'	a
2	B	b / a'
3	C	c

Scenario 2:

Priority	Surgeon	Patient
1	B	a
2	A / A'	b / a'
3	X	

Scenario 3:

Priority	Surgeon	Patient
1	A / C	b
2	B -	a'
3	A'	a / c

Fig. 4. The chart depicts a clinical application of the Ghavami Gluteal Graphic. Surgeons are able to assess and prioritize which zones require augmentation, reduction or no change. Patients can be asked the same question to determine if there are discrepancies with the surgeon's operative plan. Upper case letters are the surgeon's prioritization while lower case letters are the patient's. A (−) denotes reduction in volume for that region. An (X) through the letter indicates no change to that zone. When two letters are next to each other, they are of equal priority. Scenario 1 is an example of high fidelity between the surgeons plan and the patient's complaints while scenario 3 demonstrates a complete discrepancy.

changes from various viewpoints, surgeons are able to plan their operation and students benefit from seeing the underlying surgical roadmap that is explains how one gets certain results.

The senior author has implemented the gluteal diagram into his practice for the past 5 years. He has found that it improves patient understanding, two-way communication, and overall efficiency of the consultation. With this simple, easy to understand visual, patients confirm regional areas of excess adiposity and are able to comprehend the overall re-shaping transformation that can be expected from the S-Curve® procedure. Also, standardizing the graphic allows surgeons to compare anticipated shape changes to the end result. Analyzing practice trends to implement necessary operative adjustments will optimize results (**Fig. 5**).

Careful observation along with critical analysis is key to successful pre-operative planning. Anticipating intra-operative findings ultimately leads to outstanding aesthetic outcomes. For example, the definition, length, and lateral extent of the inferior gluteal crease foreshadows the strength and

length of the gluteal crease adhesion respectively. The depth and structure of the intergluteal sulcus is a consequence of the sacrocutaneous ligament.[9] The amount of tethered surface area between the dermis and fascia dictates the adjacent area's expansion capacity and ultimately influences the inferior lateral shape that can be achieved. The lateral depression, colloquially referred to as the "hip dip," is formed by the lateral border of the gluteus maximus, the quadratus femoris, and the insertions of the gluteus medius and vastus lateralis to the greater trochanter.[6] An anatomic dissection with simulated fat transfer found that the iliotibial band creates a boundary and marks the anterolateral extent of the buttock.[3] Meticulous examination will reveal subtle or obvious asymmetries between the two sides and any pre-existing contour deformities. Skin characteristics such as thickness and elasticity contribute to fill capacitance and longevity. All these factors influence the surgical blueprint and intra-operative decision making the surgeon must make in order to achieve optimum results. The Ghavami Gluteal Graphic allows one to recording these observations in a systematic

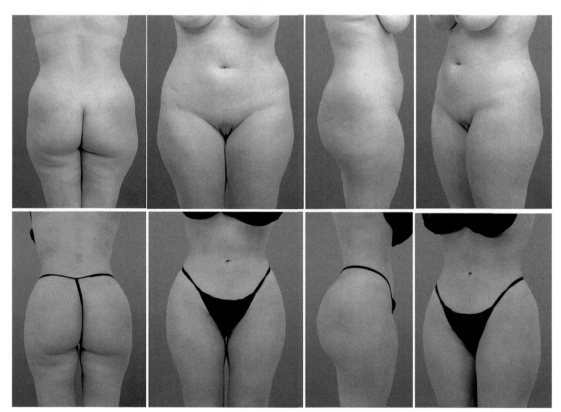

Fig. 5. This is a 29-year-old female desiring medium definition lipo-contouring of the abdomen, flanks and back. Achieving torso-buttock-thigh harmony with an S-Curve® also includes precise fat transfer to the buttock for augmentation and re-shaping. Pre-operative photographs (top row) and 1-year post-operative (bottom row).

manner and incorporate these considerations into the surgical plan.

Gluteal augmentation with fat transfer is one of the most artistic procedures in plastic surgery. Both processes, harvesting fat from areas of excess and grafting areas of deficiency to create gentle curves circumferentially demand considerable creativity and vision. Paralleling the act of commissioning artists to produce a paintings or sculpture, patients understandably exhibit a certain level of anxiety when they become the canvass and permit the surgeon to sculpt their torso. The ability to effectively communicate the anticipated end result to patients helps ease this anxiety. Visual aids and diagrams expedite this process and ensure that the patient's goals align with the surgeon's vision. Additionally, the gluteal diagram that divides the buttock into three critical parts: A, B, and C (see **Fig. 2**). A' is an adjacent subsection of territory A that represents the inferio-medial aspect which often requires particular attention and expansion. Overall, this assists the surgeon when executing the blueprint in the operating room. This enables the surgeon to sequentially concentrate their efforts on contouring a smaller area. By doing so, this operation become more manageable and once the three critical areas have been individually contoured, the overall buttock begins to take good shape. Small adjustments or maneuvers to blend the transitions between regions A, B, and C may be required but this system streamlines an artistically demanding sculpting procedure.

A recent systematic review identified 24 studies that investigated the utility and efficacy of patient information leaflets.[12] Variables considered include who provides the patient with the leaflets, supplement instead of substitute oral information provided by the physician and the specificity/generalizability of the information provided in the leaflet. While this study included data from all medical specialties, certain concepts hold validity in the plastic surgery realm. Informational visual aids and leaflets boost patient knowledge, satisfaction and play a role in their decision making. The impact was profound when this information was laid out in a concise but precise manner.[12] Concurrent with the findings, the author's diagram adds value during the consultation by supplementing the oral information provided to the patient. In addition, the advantage of the diagram is that it is simple, concise, easy to comprehend, and can be personalized to highlight certain patient specifics.

In 2018, Vartanian and colleagues published a crowdsourcing-based assessment of the ideal thigh-buttock relationship. They found that respondents preferred a wider upper thigh, creating a gentle transition from the buttocks to the legs.[13] In 2021, Mowlavi and colleagues surveyed 422 patients and reported that desired buttock shape and size varied based on age, ethnicity, and religion.[14] Hispanics and African Americans preferred larger sizes with emphasis on the lower pole compared to Caucasians. Older patients and Muslim respondents tended to prefer a smaller sized buttock. The authors subsequently converted the survey to an "Assessment Tool" and hypothesized that this would serve as a guide for evaluation, preoperative discussion, and intra-operative execution.[15] The charts are rather cumbersome to implement in a clinical setting as they have created over 30 caricatures by varying the waist-to-hip ratio, area of maximal projection and anterioposterior versus lateral views. This study ultimately highlights the need for developing a simple diagram that allows the surgeon and patient to communicate their thoughts efficiently. We believe that the graphic meets these criteria; it is easy to use by surgeons, easy to understand by patients, and generalizable yet adaptable to individuals.

LIMITATIONS

A limitation is that this is designed specifically for gluteal lipo-augmentation candidates. Massive weight-loss patients or those with significant skin laxity/ptosis, would benefit more from a buttock lift. The approach and design for excisional procedures differs from volume re-distribution procedures. Unlike image morphing programs that use the patient's own photos to manipulate curves and adjust sizes, this standardized graphic serves as the foundation for the consultation where a surgeon's superimposed drawings/markings illustrate the anticipated changes from this procedure. Surgeon familiarity with the diagram ultimately saves time as is eliminates the need to upload photographs into computer programs and precisely adjust the bodies outline to reflect changes in gluteal shape. Also, certain surgeons fear that patients will view morphed images as accurate renditions of the expected surgical result and hold the surgeon accountable to reproducing the exact shaped that was promised. Ultimately, the diagramming method offers a buffer these expectations and protects the surgeon.

SUMMARY

The graphic designed by the senior author is simple, effective, and appreciated by both the surgeon and patient. The outline of the buttock shape, gentle curves from the upper back to the thighs and relative ideal proportions helps patients contrast to their current body shape. Additionally, by creating subsections A, B, C and A′, patients are able to better comprehend which particular areas need the volume and contour adjustments. Particularly in instances where donor site adiposity is limited, the Ghavami Gluteal Graphic system is an effective way for the surgeon and patient to agree upon which area ought to be prioritized. Moreover, this diagram coupled with the consultation notes/mark-ups, provides the surgeon with a useful intra-operative blueprint.

CLINICS CARE POINTS

Pearls

- A simple, easy to understand graphic that enhances a patient's understanding of the various aspects involved in re-shaping the torso and gluteal areas during gluteal augmentation procedures.
- Dividing the buttock into the four critical areas (Areas A, A′, B and C in Figure 2) allows the surgeon to temporarily concentrate efforts in order to optimize overall contours and to prioritize which areas fat will be transferred to in cases of donor site scarcity.

Pitfalls

- Misalignment in patient expectations and the surgeon's artistic vision compromises satisfaction and clinical outcomes.
- Transcribing the visualized circumferential contours and areas of excess versus areas of deficiency on two-dimensional diagrams requires practice and experience.

DISCLOSURE

Dr. A. Ghavami: Royalties from Thieme Pub, QMP and Consultant/Advisor for MTF Inc, Advisor/Marketing Partner InMode Inc.

ACKNOWLEDGMENTS

The authors appreciate Joseph H. Talbot, MD, for his artistic talents in creating the illustrations.

REFERENCES

1. Centeno RF, Sood A, Young VL. Clinical anatomy in aesthetic gluteal contouring. Clin Plast Surg 2018; 45(2):145–57.
2. Mendieta CG. Classification system for gluteal evaluation. Clin Plast Surg 2006;33(3):333–46.
3. Frojo G, Halani SH, Pessa JE, et al. Deep subcutaneous gluteal fat compartments : anatomy and clinical implications deep subcutaneous gluteal fat compartments : anatomy and clinical implications. Aesthetic Surg J 2022;00(0):1–8.
4. Cansancao AL, Conde-Green A, David JA, et al. Subcutaneous-only gluteal fat grafting : a prospective study of the long-term results with ultrasoound analysis. Plast Reconstr Surg 2018;143(2):447–51.
5. Mendieta CG, Sood A. Classification system for gluteal evaluation: revisited. Clin Plast Surg 2018; 45(2):159–77.
6. Ghavami A, Villanueva NL, Amirlak B. Gluteal ligamentous anatomy and its implication in safe buttock augmentation. Plast Reconstr Surg 2018;142(2): 363–71.
7. Del Vecchio D, Wall S. Expansion vibration lipofilling: a new technique in large-volume fat transplantation. Plast Reconstr Surg 2018;141(5):639e–49e.
8. Abboud M, Geeroms M, El Hajj H, et al. Improving the female silhouette and gluteal projection: an anatomy-based, safe, and harmonious approach through liposuction, suspension loops, and moderate lipofilling. Aesthetic Surg J 2021;41(4):474–89.
9. Gonzalez R, Gonzalez R. Intramuscular gluteal augmentation: the XYZ method. Clin Plast Surg 2018;45(2):217–23.
10. Dekkers T, Melles M, Mathijssen NMC, et al. Tailoring the orthopaedic consultation: how perceived patient characteristics influence surgeons' communication. Patient Educ Counsel 2018;101(3):428–38.
11. Yahanda AT, Lafaro KJ, Spolverato G, et al. A systematic review of the factors that patients use to choose their surgeon. World J Surg 2016;40(1): 45–55.
12. Sustersic M, Gauchet A, Foote A, et al. How best to use and evaluate Patient Information Leaflets given during a consultation: a systematic review of literature reviews. Health Expect 2017;20(4):531–42.
13. Vartanian E, Gould DJ, Hammoudeh ZS, et al. The ideal thigh: a crowdsourcing-based assessment of ideal thigh aesthetic and implications for gluteal fat grafting. Aesthetic Surg J 2018;38(8):861–9.
14. Mowlavi A, Berri M, Talle A, et al. Objectifying high-definition Brazilian buttock lift results using the buttock assessment tool. Plast Reconstr Surg 2021;148(5):727E–34E.
15. Mowlavi A, Sin Z, Sahami C, et al. Optimizing Brazilian buttock lift results using the BBL assessment tool. Aesthetic Plast Surg 2022. https://doi.org/10.1007/s00266-022-03120-1. ePub.

Aesthetic Ideals of the Female Buttocks
Concepts and Techniques

Stefan Danilla, MD, MSc[a],*, Diana Micheli, MD[b]

KEYWORDS

• Buttocks • Anatomy • Ideal • Model • Female • Gluteal sculpting • Gluteal reshaping

KEY POINTS

- Understanding the tridimensional artistic anatomy of the back, pelvis, and thighs is essential for successful gluteal surgery.
- Ethnic differences play a significant role in determining the ideal aesthetic outcomes in gluteal procedures, and surgeons must consider and respect these variations.
- Individualization of treatment is crucial in gluteal surgery to meet the specific needs and preferences of each patient.
- Communication and collaboration between the surgeon and the patient are vital in determining the desired aesthetic goals and achieving satisfactory outcomes.
- Anatomic knowledge, cultural sensitivity, and a comprehensive approach are essential for achieving natural and aesthetically pleasing results in gluteal enhancement procedures.

HISTORIC PERSPECTIVE

Throughout the annals of civilization, the female gluteal area has remained an enduring symbol of beauty and attraction.[1] Artists and scholars alike have dedicated their talents and studies to unraveling the intricate anatomy of the gluteal region for more than 2 millennia (Fig. 1). Its allure transcends time and cultural boundaries, captivating the imagination and inspiring admiration across generations.

Traditionally, the teaching of anatomy in medical schools and surgical residencies has focused on the layers of tissue, blood supply, and innervation of various body structures. However, the three-dimensionality and intricate interplay of the gluteal region's structures have often been overlooked. This oversight fails to fully convey the complexity and beauty of this remarkable anatomic landscape.

BUTTOCK ANATOMY AND CHARACTERISTICS

The gluteal area is not simply a singular structure but rather a complex composition of various elements, including bones, muscles, subcutaneous fat, and skin. In their contributions, Cuenca-Guerra and Quezada, Mendieta, and De la Peña and colleagues[2–4] have shed light on the understanding of aesthetic traits that define a beautiful buttock. These traits can be summarized as follows.

1. *Bony Structure*: The shape of the pelvis plays a significant role in influencing the perception of beauty. Four distinct pelvis shapes have been identified: A, V, circular, and square. Among these, the "A" shape and circular shape are considered the most aesthetically pleasing.
2. *Gluteus Maximus Muscle*: The development of the gluteus maximus muscle greatly contributes to the overall aesthetics of the buttocks. Athletic, well-developed muscle mass in this region enhances the projection and shape of the buttocks.
3. *Subcutaneous Fat Compartment*: The distribution of subcutaneous fat in the gluteal region is an important factor in achieving the desired aesthetic proportions. Proper fat distribution

[a] Cirujano Plástico Magíster en Epidemiología Clínica, Clínica AUREA, Santiago, Chile; [b] Equipo de Cirugia Plástica, Pontificia Universidad Catolica, Santiago, Chile
* Corresponding author.
E-mail addresses: stefan@drdanilla.cl; drstefandanilla@gmail.com

Clin Plastic Surg 50 (2023) 533–540
https://doi.org/10.1016/j.cps.2023.06.002

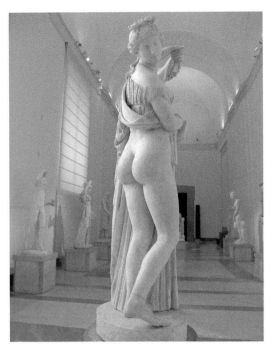

Fig. 1. The goddess of beauty, Aphrodite Kallipygos or Callipygian Venus. (*From* Venere Callipige. Museo archeologica nazionale di Napoli. Collezione Farnese. [https:// commons.wikimedia.org/wiki/File:Venere_Callipige_ Napoli.jpg] by ho visto nina volare. September 10, 2012. Public Domain.)

helps create a harmonious contour and volume in the buttocks.
4. *Skin*: The quality of the skin in the gluteal area also plays a role in buttock aesthetics. Elasticity and turgidity of the skin contribute to a smooth, youthful appearance.

In addition, it is crucial to consider surrounding anatomic structures that influence the overall aesthetic proportions of the buttocks. The waist, lower back, sacral area, and thighs should be taken into account to achieve a natural and harmonious result. For instance, an imbalance whereby the buttocks are significantly larger compared with thin thighs, often created by isolated fat grafting to the buttocks, is referred to as the "ant deformity." This term is used to describe the unnatural appearance that results from such disproportions (**Fig. 2**A–D).

THE ARTISTIC VISION AND PERCEPTIONS

To gain a comprehensive understanding of the superficial tridimensionality of the female posterior, it proves useful to approach the study from an artistic perspective.[5] Complexity amplifies as lines in the first dimension progress to shapes in the second

dimension and ultimately to volume in the third dimension. The intricacies involved in appreciating volumetric size and symmetry required for plastic surgery demands a high level of architectural and artistic vision.

In **Fig. 3**A, a sketch depicts the silhouette of a woman with a beautiful body, showcasing the ideal proportions of the waist, hips, buttocks, and thighs. These harmonious proportions create a visually pleasing and balanced appearance.

To further enhance contrast and shadowing, artificial lines are introduced in **Fig. 3**B to emphasize major muscle groups and create a sense of depth and definition. These lines include the posterior belly of the deltoid, a midline from the interscapular region to the L4-5 level, the lateral border of the paravertebral muscles, the posterior superior iliac spine (also known as the dimples of Venus), and the insertion of the gluteus major along the inferolateral border of the sacrum and iliac crests.

By blending these major lines, valleys, and muscle groups together, a sense of tridimensionality is achieved, as depicted in **Fig. 3**C. A complete understanding of anatomy allows the surgeon to sculpt the subcutaneous fat, either by removing it or by adding volume through techniques like fat grafting or implants. These interventions enable the surgeon to create or accentuate the desired anatomic features.

GLUTEAL CONTOURING: THE SURGEON-ARTIST

When applying these artistic concepts to the clinical setting, as shown in **Fig. 3**D, surgeons can greatly enhance the outcomes of gluteal surgeries. Taking into account the interplay of lines, valleys, and muscle groups, as well as the individual patient's unique anatomy, surgeons can achieve results that align with the patient's aesthetic goals and natural contours.

This approach, combining artistic principles with surgical expertise, empowers surgeons to create outcomes that harmonize with the multidimensional beauty of the female posterior.

In **Fig. 4**A, the targeted areas for liposuction of the superficial fat are marked in green. These areas include the posterior belly of the deltoid, the midline, the insertion of the gluteus major muscle in the sacrum, as well as the posterior iliac spine and iliac crest. By selectively removing excess fat in these regions, the surgeon can enhance the definition and contour of the posterior body, resulting in a more sculpted and aesthetically pleasing appearance. Liposuction techniques allow for precise fat removal while preserving the underlying natural curves and proportions of the gluteal area.[6,7]

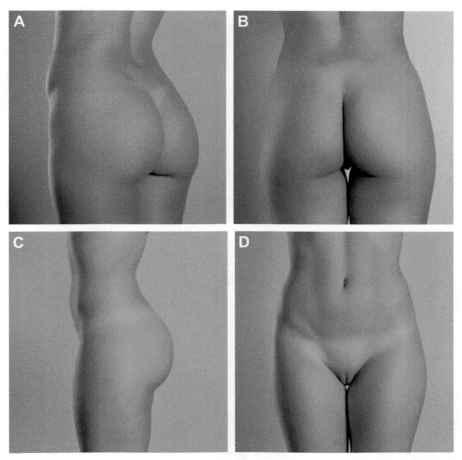

Fig. 2. (*A–D*) Anterior, posterior, lateral, and posterior oblique views of a woman, without surgical intervention. This demonstrates aesthetically pleasing gluteal contours with harmonious proportions relative to the torso and thighs.

To reveal the underlying anatomy of the muscles, it is important to remove the deep fat in the posterior arm and flanks. This can be achieved through liposuction techniques that target the deeper layers of fat. By selectively removing the deep fat deposits, surgeons expose the contours and definition of the underlying muscles, such as the triceps in the posterior arm region. This not only enhances the muscular appearance but also contributes to a more sculpted and toned overall aesthetic. By addressing the deep fat in these areas, the surgeon can achieve a harmonious balance between muscle definition and body contouring (**Fig. 4**B).

Preserving fat over the paravertebral muscles can indeed contribute to enhancing the muscular appearance of the lower and middle back. The layer of fat over these muscles can provide a subtle amount of padding that accentuates the underlying muscle contours, creating a more defined and sculpted appearance. By selectively removing fat in other areas while preserving volume over the

paravertebral muscles, the surgeon can achieve a harmonious balance between muscle definition and overall body contouring.

In the buttock area, the surgeon has the option to improve its appearance by adding volume through either implants or fat grafting, depending on their preferences and the desired results of the patient.[6–11] Implants can provide a predictable and controlled increase in buttock volume, whereas fat grafting involves harvesting fat from other areas of the body and injecting it into the buttocks to achieve the desired shape and fullness. Both techniques have their advantages and considerations, and the choice depends on factors such as the patient's anatomy,[12,13] aesthetic goals, and the surgeon's expertise.

Fig. 4C illustrates the potential outcome of these procedures, showcasing the enhanced muscular appearance of the lower and middle back, as well as the improved volume and shape of the buttock area. However, it is important to note that individual results may vary, and a comprehensive evaluation

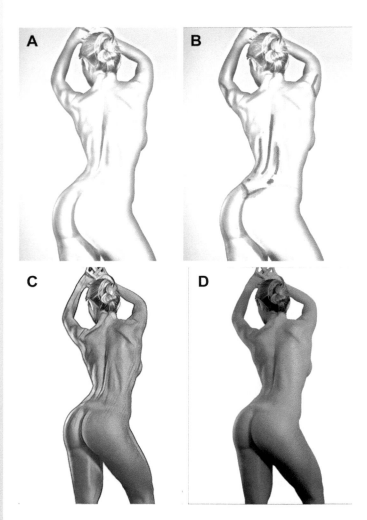

Fig. 3. (A) Silhouette of an athletic woman from a posterior-oblique view. (B) The same drawing with additional sketch marks to highlight transitions between muscular groups. (C) Muscular volumes in 3D can be appreciated in this black and white drawing of the athletic woman. (D) The actual photograph of an athletic woman.

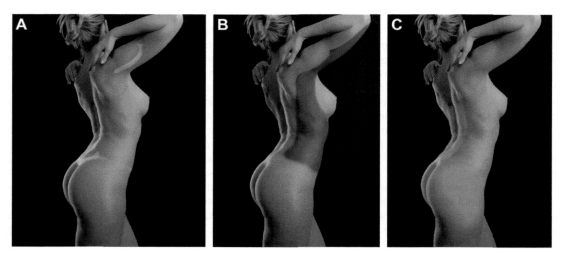

Fig. 4. (A) Negative zones, highlighted in green, are accentuated by meticulous superficial liposuction. (B) The purple depicts areas where deep liposuction is performed for debulking. (C) The red depicts areas that are frequently augmented with fat grafting or implants.

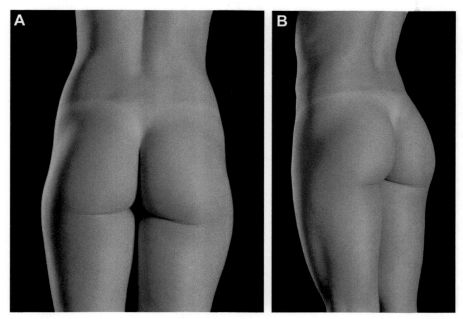

Fig. 5. (*A, B*) Posterior and posterior-oblique photographs of an athletic woman that demonstrate a natural transition zone between gluteus mayor and medius muscles.

and personalized approach are necessary to achieve the desired outcome.

THE LATERAL DEPRESSION OF THE BUTTOCKS

The lateral aspect of the buttock can vary depending on patient-specific characteristics, such as degree of muscularity, ethnicity, age, body mass index, and history of weight fluctuations. In some women, particularly those with hypertrophy of the hip muscles and a minimal amount of subcutaneous fat in the hip area, a prominent lateral depression or concavity may be observed. This can create a distinct contour in the outer part of the buttock, giving it a more athletic appearance.

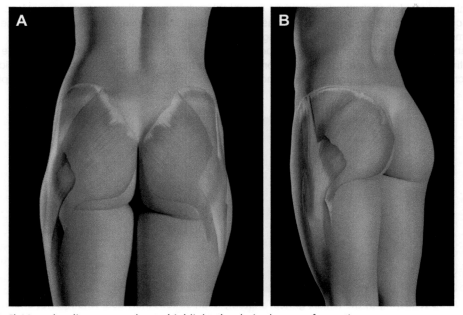

Fig. 6. (*A, B*) Muscular diagram overlay to highlight the desired areas of negative space.

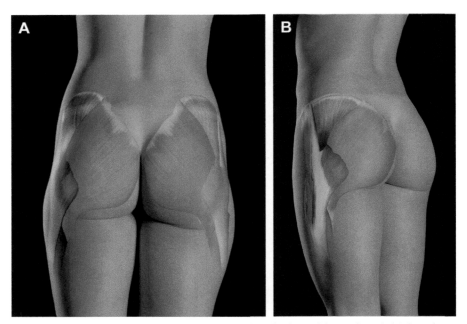

Fig. 7. (*A, B*) The green highlight serves as a general guideline for lateral buttock and thigh sculpting to accentuate an athletic appearance.

The presence of a lateral depression is influenced by factors such as the individual's muscle development, distribution of subcutaneous fat, and overall body composition. Some individuals naturally have more prominent hip muscles, which can contribute to the appearance of a lateral depression. In addition, ethnic variations in body shape and fat distribution can also play a role.

For patients who desire to address or enhance the lateral aspect of their buttocks, surgical options, such as fat grafting or targeted muscle enhancement, can be considered.[14] Fat grafting involves harvesting fat from other areas of the body and injecting it strategically into the lateral depression to create a smoother and more rounded

contour when viewed from the posterior-anterior direction. In cases where muscle enhancement is desired, specific exercises and targeted strength training can be used to develop and shape the hip muscles, resulting in a more balanced and harmonious overall buttock appearance (**Fig. 5**A, B).

The presence of a lateral depression in the buttock area can be attributed to several factors, including the bulkiness of the gluteus major muscle, gluteus medius muscle, tensor fasciae latae muscle, and the depression caused by the iliotibial tract.

Addressing the lateral depression in the buttock area may involve a combination of surgical techniques, such as targeted muscle sculpting, fat

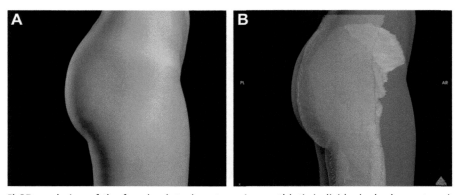

Fig. 8. (*A, B*) 3D rendering of the female gluteal anatomy in an athletic individual who has not undergone surgical interventions.

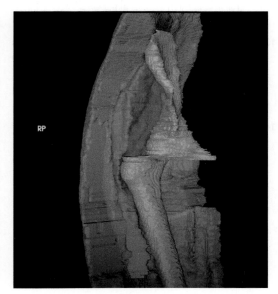

Fig. 9. An axial view of a 3D MRI rendering depicting an even amount of subcutaneous thickness over the gluteal area.

grafting, or liposuction. The goal is to achieve a more balanced and harmonious contour by reducing the prominence of certain muscles and adding volume where needed (see **Fig. 5**; **Figs. 6 and 7**).

Also important to notice is that, in athletic women, the thickness of the subcutaneous fat over the gluteus major is even and does not enlarge over the muscle, and the shape of the buttocks is mainly determined by the bony structure and the volume of all the pelvic muscles. An MRI, three-dimensional (3D) reconstruction of the fat layer over the muscles, gluteus major muscle, and bones of the pelvis and femur shows the distribution of the anatomic structures in a buttocks model (**Fig. 8A, B**). An even thickness of subcutaneous fat can be appreciated throughout the entirety of the posterior pelvis (**Fig. 9**).

SUMMARY

In summary, in order to adequately understand gluteal surgery, the plastic surgeon must be familiar with the concepts of tridimensional artistic anatomy of the back, pelvis, and thighs. Several techniques exist to improve the appearance of each specific region, and it is crucial to consider the ethnic and sociocultural differences of the patient and the surgeon. By recognizing and respecting these variations, as well as individualizing each treatment approach, the surgeon can achieve optimal results that align with the patient's preferences and cultural background.

CLINICS CARE POINTS

- Understand the importance of ethnic differences in determining ideal aesthetic outcomes and respect cultural variations.
- Individualize treatment based on each patient's preferences and needs.
- Foster effective communication and collaboration between the surgeon and the patient to determine desired aesthetic goals.
- Use comprehensive anatomic knowledge, cultural sensitivity, and a personalized approach for successful gluteal enhancement procedures.
- Communicate openly with the patient, ensuring their understanding in order to align expected outcomes of the procedure.
- Use three-dimensional artistic anatomy knowledge of the back, pelvis, thigh and buttocks to guide surgical techniques and achieve natural-looking results.

DISCLOSURE

The author has nothing to disclose.

REFERENCES

1. Gonzalez R. Gluteoplastía. Editorial Indexa; Edición: 2nd (2012).
2. Cuenca-Guerra R, Quezada J. What makes buttocks beautiful? a review and classification of the determinants of gluteal beauty and the surgical techniques to achieve them. Aesthetic Plast Surg 2004;28(5):340–7.
3. Mendieta CG. Classification system for gluteal evaluation. Clin Plast Surg 2006;33(3):333–46.
4. De la Peña JA, Rubio OV, Cano JP, et al. Subfascial gluteal augmentation. Clin Plast Surg 2006;33(3): 405–22.
5. Danilla S, Troncoso E, Jara R, et al. What makes a beautiful buttock beautiful? a case-control study comparing buttocks models versus normal women by magnetic resonance imaging, photography and anthropometry. Aesthetic Plast Surg 2022. https://doi.org/10.1007/s00266-022-03222-w.
6. Mendieta C, Stuzin JM. Gluteal augmentation and enhancement of the female silhouette. Plast Reconstr Surg 2018;141(2):306–11.
7. Del Vecchio D, Wall S Jr. Expansion vibration lipofilling: a new technique in large-volume fat transplantation. Plast Reconstr Surg 2018;141:639e–49e.

8. Gonzalez R, Gonzalez R. Intramuscular gluteal augmentation: the XYZ method. Clin Plast Surg 2018;45(2):217–23.

9. Gonzalez R. Augmentation gluteoplasty: the XYZ method. Aesthetic Plast Surg 2004;28:417–25.

10. Gonzalez R. Gluteal implants: the "XYZ" intramuscular method. Aesthet Surg J 2010;30(2):256–64.

11. Aslani A, Del Vecchio DA. Composite buttock augmentation. Plast Reconstr Surg 2019;144(6):1312–21.

12. Danilla S. Espesor normal del músculo glúteo mayor en mujeres chilenas. Una guía para el aumento de glúteo con implantes. Rev Chil Cir 2016;68(6): 427–32.

13. Multi Society Gluteal Fat Grafting Task Force issues safety advisory urging practitioners to reevaluate technique. Aesthet Surg J. Available at: http://www.jsprs.or.jp/member/committee/module/15/pdf/20180202_Statement.pdf. Accessed September 20, 2018.

14. Cárdenas-Camarena L, Durán H. Improvement of the gluteal contour. Clin Plast Surg 2018;45(2): 237–47.

Combining Gluteal Shaping with High-Definition Liposuction
New Concepts and Techniques

Alfredo E. Hoyos Ariza, MD[a],*, Mauricio Perez Pachon, MD[b]

KEYWORDS

- Body contouring • Anatomy • High-definition liposuction • Gluteal contouring • Fat grafting
- Buttock aesthetics

KEY POINTS

- Buttock aesthetics are not only male/female-based anymore.
- New aesthetic trends are based on binary and non-binary appealing preferences, which the surgeon must acknowledge before attempting gluteal liposculpture.
- Fat Grafting to the buttocks' area is not just volume enhancement and equalization but also 4-dimensional projection and structural support for long lasting results.
- Dynamic Definition Liposculpture enhances the volume perception and the natural slim/athletic contour of both the lower extremity and the lower back, which boosts up the projection of the buttock and reducing the need of massive volume lipoinjection.
- Most complications after gluteal reshaping procedures can be either prevented or acknowledged with proper planning and execution.

BACKGROUND

The appearance and projection of the gluteal region are considered an evolutionary adaptation to erect and bipedal posture.[1] Gender, culture, and geography influence the aesthetic standards of this anatomic region.[2,3] Objective definition of a beauty buttock includes contour uniformity, adequate projection of the mid and upper third, as well as softness, skin smoothness, and elasticity, while peri-gluteal fat accumulation has been shown to distort the ideal gluteal shape.[4] Four variables interact to give the buttocks their appearance: underlying bone framework, gluteus maximus muscle, subcutaneous fat, and skin.[5] Out of these variables, *subcutaneous fat* is considered the most important and susceptible to

intervention. It contributes to buttock projection and impacts the framing over which the gluteus muscle rests.[1,5]

Artistic Anatomy

Both High Definition (HDL) and Dynamic Definition Liposculpture (HD2) incorporate lipoplasty techniques for the whole body and not an individual region. However, in this article, we will be extrapolating concepts from HDL and HD2 to the buttock area. Gluteal shapes are defined according to the amount of fat located in 3 different anatomic sites: the upper lateral hip, the most protruding point in the lateral thigh, and the lateral mid-buttock. The resulting shapes are square, A-shaped, V-shaped, and round.[5] Variations in

[a] Dhara Clinic, Private Practice, Av Carrera 15 #83-33 Suite 203, Bogota, Colombia; [b] Private Practice, Rochester, MN, USA
* Corresponding author.
E-mail address: alhoyos@gmail.com

Clin Plastic Surg 50 (2023) 541–552
https://doi.org/10.1016/j.cps.2023.06.008
0094-1298/23/© 2023 Elsevier Inc. All rights reserved.

subcutaneous fat distribution take place during age, weight gain, or loss processes, and differ according to sex and ethnicity.[1] Indeed, android and gynoid body types depend on gluteal fat distribution. The lateral border of the gluteus is continuous with the anterior thigh and pelvis. As women age, they tend to develop a centralized fat distribution pattern with the greatest differences at the waist and mid-trochanter level compared to younger women, buttocks increase their height and lengthen the intergluteal crease and intergluteal fold.[1] Similar changes are caused by weight gain. Previously, "ideal" female buttocks had to have the shape of a hemisphere whereby the only defined edge would be the inferior-medial zone whereas the other borders would smoothly diffuse within the leg and torso. Comparatively for men, a square shape during resting position (standing) and a butterfly shape with active contraction, altogether with sharp muscle borders and gluteus medius definition would be the most accurate approach. We strongly believe that the lower back and the hamstrings are both highly determinant in defining this round/squared shape of the gluteus; however, recent trends of society towards avoiding binary limitations of many different human philosophies have also impacted the aesthetic surgery field in the good way of broadening our perspective of HDL. In effect, prior aesthetic concepts can be merged to achieve not only a male or female *façade* but rather variable degree of definition in HD2. To note, male gluteal shape is mainly determined by the underlying gluteus maximus with little adipose tissue, with sharp edges producing a distinctive slim and muscular appearance. Due to hormonal receptors and estrogen related-fat deposits, men do not accumulate significant amounts of adipose tissue in the gluteal area but rather in the central abdomen and torso compared to women, who usually accumulate fat over the hips, legs and arms. These gender differences are a determinant for the surgical technique, aesthetic goals, and postoperative recovery.

Aesthetic zones of the gluteal area

We described 4 anatomical zones for men, and although they are quite related to those from women, the surgeon must acknowledge that for the latter such sharp limits ultimately blend with each other to create a continuum of body silhouette (**Figs. 1** and **2**). Therefore.

- *Zone 1* (flank) extends from the posterior lower rib cage margin to the superior iliac crest and lateral border of the erector spinae muscles. This region blends with the superior

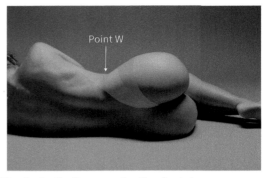

Fig. 1. Aesthetic zones for the feminine appearance of the gluteal area. Red zone: lateral and above the superior pole of the glutes. Green zone: Supragluteal flank area. Point W: Most pronounced limit of indentation over the waist.

gluteal area in women (a.k.a. *Red zone*) and should be named the supragluteal flank area (a.k.a. *Green zone*) whereby thorough liposuction will help to define the waistline (point W).

- *Zone 2* or Central zone is subdivided into 2 areas: the rhomboid of the sacrum (rhomboid of Michaelis) and the erector spinae muscles. The appearance of an adipose pad over the sacral prominence is possible, particularly in overweight and obese patients. This zone has virtually the same configuration for women.

- *Zone 3* or Gluteal zone is subdivided into the following 3 areas: Gluteus maximus, Gluteus medius, and Trochanteric depression. The gluteus maximus is dominant and contributes to the glute convexity, particularly in slim

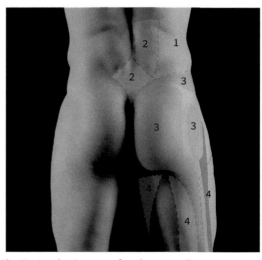

Fig. 2. Aesthetic zones for the masculine appearance of the gluteal area. Zones 1-4.

individuals. A depression over the posterior superior iliac spines is created by the lack of muscle coverage of this bony structure, which should not be sharply defined in women, but actually blended (*green* and *red zones*). The inferior medial border of the gluteus maximus is covered by gluteal fat and provides volume to the medial region of the infra-gluteal fold. The muscle bulk of the gluteus maximus (posteriorly) and the gluteus medius (superiorly) create a "C"-shaped concavity with the greater trochanter. This depression is important to keep the masculine appearance as it is more pronounced in men than women. To note, a mild to moderate definition of this area will help women to achieve a more athletic and muscular appearance, while a soft blending will result in a more delicate gluteal area for men. Additionally, the gluteus medius can be fat grafted to increase its lateral projection and both the athletic and masculine appearance of the buttock, however, we do not consider it necessary for women.

- *Zone 4* or Infra-gluteal zone is subdivided into 4 areas: Adductors, Biceps femoris, Iliotibial tract, and Vastus lateralis. Above the iliotibial tract, Tensor fascia latae muscle fuses superiorly with the upper portion of the gluteus medius and, eventually, the flank.

Infragluteal fold
Recent cadaveric-based studies have changed the anatomic standpoints of the structure of the Superficial Fascia System (SFS) at the gluteal region.[6] In fact, there is no such thing as a uniform structure but rather a genetically predisposed configuration of both the dermic and fat components of the SFS at the infragluteal fold (IFF). Its length and toughness will depend on: 1- Number of fibers and disposition of the supporting connective tissue coming from its origin at the sacrum; and 2- The variable adipose component that will ultimately blend laterally with the SFS of the thigh (**Fig. 3**). Peri-gluteal fat below the inferior gluteal fold deserves a special consideration. What we all know as "banana roll" is actually a unique female anatomical subdermal configuration below the inferior gluteal fold that resembles a reel. The interplay of the posterior fascia latae of the thigh with the cutis-dependent SFS of the gluteal fold will derive in a wider, thinner or even absent roll. Therefore, this zone cannot be over-resected as it may alter the gluteal surrounding and end up with a fake or prosthetic appearance, rather than a natural one. On the other side, there is a growing amount of non-binary patients who would prefer a different body profile including their buttocks.

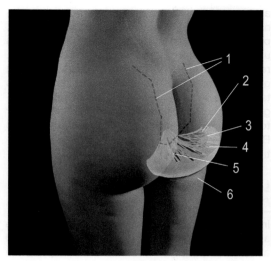

Fig. 3. Structure of the Infragluteal fold and its relationship with the superficial fascia system of the thigh. (*Adapted from* Si L, Li Z, Fu L, et al. Gluteal Fold: Cadaveric Dissection of the Superficial Fascial System in the Buttock and Anatomy-based Gluteal Liposculpture [published online ahead of print, 2023 May 22]. Plast Reconstr Surg. 2023;10.1097/PRS.0000000000010723.)

Some of them stick with the usual gender-based approach, while others do want an "in-between" pattern. Regarding body feminization, the goal is to recreate the well-known hourglass feminine body shape, which includes a low waist-to-hip ratio (approximately 0,6/0,7), compared to that of the traditional V-shaped male figure. In that sense, "in-between" pattern for women would be a more square-shaped buttock, while a rounder shape would be for men. In fact, women who are actually very fit and muscular usually prefer a soft definition of the trochanteric depression (which is an actual feature of male buttock reshaping) to improve the muscular appearance of their glutes.[7]

Current gluteal definition procedures include the use of implants, autologous fat transfer, excisional procedures, autologous gluteal augmentation with tissue flaps and liposuction. Implants have a slightly higher incidence of complications compared to that from fat grafting; yet, hybrid surgeries show very promising results for those patients who would require massive-volume lipoinjections.[8-12] Additionally, even if most of the patients who undergo these procedures are females, there has been an increase in the number of men who pursue aesthetic body contour surgery, which has challenged plastic surgeons to develop male-specific approaches. New approaches to gluteal contour reshaping and enhancement in men focus on the desired shape at rest and during contraction, associated to dynamic definition body contouring principles, providing a natural look aligned with the patient's underlying anatomy. Del Vecchio and colleagues, recently published a practice advisory regarding gluteal fat grafting. The recommendations of this task force include the utilization of ultrasound-guided documentation of cannula placement prior to and during fat injection, and the limitation of 3 BBL cases as a maximum amount of total operative cases per day.[13]

SURGICAL TECHNIQUES
Preoperative Markings

In preparation for the contouring procedure, the areas for deep liposuction in women are marked as follows: the flanks, the sacral fat pad, the hips, and the lateral and medial thighs. The sacral dimples are marked for pure framing, these define the basic definition markings. The roll below the gluteal fold is also marked, as it will determine the inferior projection of the gluteus. Also, we should consider that the marks for superficial liposuction are set according to the definition degree desired. In men fat deposits in the gluteal area are marked for resection (**Fig. 4**).

Patient must be in the standing position for special markings. The superior gluteal edge is identified following the shape of the iliac bone to the anterior iliac crest. Subsequently, the posterior lower rib edge and the lateral border of the erector spinae are marked, delimitating the flank zone whereby the fat can be freely removed. To note, either rib corticotomy or resection can be done to improve the waist definition in both men and women. In female patients we must identify the maximum point of indentation (PMI) in the waistline and trace a line to the upper limit of the intergluteal crease (UIC), and then a line from this point to the superior iliac crest. The triangle area created is the first green zone (zone for free fat extraction). Next, the trochanteric depression is marked on the lateral side and a line is traced from its upper limit to the top of the inter-gluteal crease creating a triangular area (red zone) for complete (deep and superficial) fat removal. This marking is common for both male and female patients. The gluteus maximus upper limits are then marked in contraction (**Fig. 5**).

For both male and female patients, the inferior gluteal area is marked and divided into four zones by placing a vertical line through the center of the gluteus maximus and a horizontal line through the inferior gluteal fold. We mark negative spaces according to gender. In males a total of 3 negative areas (targeted for smooth definition and carving

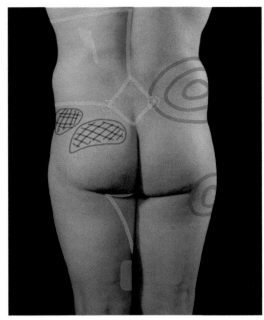

Fig. 4. Preoperative gluteal markings of the male patient. Adipose deposits are marked with blue. Negative spaces are marked with green. Adhesion zones are marked with red, while zones for fat grafting are marked with purple.

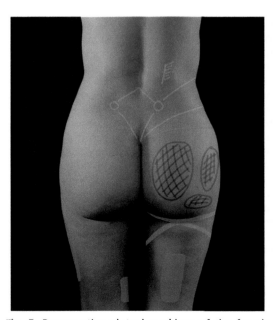

Fig. 5. Preoperative gluteal markings of the female patient. Negative spaces (*green*) and adhesion zones (*red*) are marked together with the zones for fat grafting (*purple*).

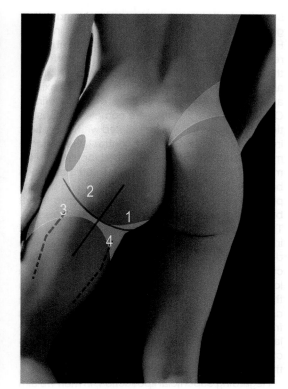

Fig. 6. Gluteal specifics of the inferior zone of the female buttock and its relationship with the thigh.

out the fat for body sculpting are marked: the proximal portion of the inner thigh, the red zone, and the trochanteric depression).[14] The adhesion zone of the middle third of the inner thigh is marked in order to avoid deep liposuction over this area. If absolutely necessary, just a soft and smooth superficial liposuction can be performed in this area. Lateral to the infra-gluteal midpoint, the border of the gluteus is identified by grasping the posterior thigh muscles and rotating them externally to identify extra fat on the lateral buttocks which can be shifted or removed by smooth liposuction.

In women, we divide the inferior gluteal area into 4 major negative spaces according to the mid-gluteal point (**Fig. 6**).

- Zone 1: Inferior-medial gluteal area must form an acute angle to recreate a round-like buttock. It forms a continuum in the midline with the intergluteal groove.
- Zone 2: Lower external gluteal area forms a transition between the lateral buttock and the external facet of the thigh. A soft definition towards the inferior edge of the trochanteric depression and a soft blending are both mandatory to avoid an unnatural appearance.
- Zone 3: Proximal inner thigh confluences with *Zone 1* to recreate a round buttock and follow the infragluteal fold. It is important to recall that the inner thigh is divided in thirds; the middle is an adhesion zone, which contains only superficial fat, so over resection should be avoided in this area. The upper-inner thigh holds a high stem-cell concentration and is safe for both deep and superficial liposuction.
- Zone 4: Outer thigh is extended from the lateral portion of the gluteal area (*Zone 2*) to the lateral tight. It usually requires deep thorough liposuction to remove all extra fat at the lateral hip but blending upwards with the trochanteric depression and downwards with the lateral thigh.

Women looking for a more masculine appearance will require a sharper definition of a shadow behind the iliotibial tract (soft trochanteric depression). In the contrary, men looking for a more feminine appearance require a round buttock at the trochanteric depression and a soft transition with the gluteus medius.

Intraoperative procedures
Patient is placed in the prone position. Incisions are performed at the midpoint over the infragluteal fold on each side and at the inter-gluteal crease. We follow the classic 3-step process

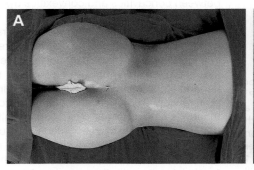
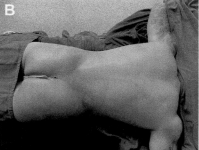

Fig. 7. Muscular definition of the lower back and its continuum with the buttocks in a female (*A*) and a male (*B*) patient. To note, no fat grafting was required for this purpose.

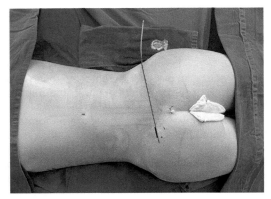

Fig. 8. Long curved cannula to reach the gluteal contour, including the trochanteric depression, the red and green zones.

(infiltration, emulsification, lipoaspiration) for Liposuction and then perform selective fat grafting. Infiltration is made with saline (1000 mL) combined with a 1:1000 ratio of 1% of lidocaine (10 mL) and epinephrine (1 mL) fat emulsification is achieved using VASER Lipo® system with a 3.7 mm 2-ringed probe and a 2.9 mm 3-ringed probe for the flank area and the thigh respectively. Once the emulsification (step 2) is complete, we proceed with liposuction.

We start liposuction in the deep layer with a 4-mm straight Mercedes cannula. In males, this

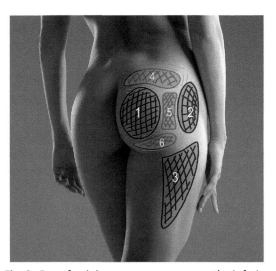

Fig. 9. For a feminine appearance, we use the inferior gluteal fold to inject two big adipose grafts for AP[1] and lateral[2] projection respectively. Then we place a small superficial graft at the gluteal pillar,[3] which will support the thigh and will improve the transition with the lateral thigh (optional). The buttock upper pole,[4] the supra fold area[6] and in-between zones 1 and 2[5] we place small superficial grafts that will smooth the transitions between big grafts.[1,2]

step is started over the lower back and upper gluteal area via the inter-gluteal crease incision. Fat lipoaspiration from the lower and lateral gluteal region and from the inner thigh is performed through the infra-gluteal midpoint incision bilaterally. Then, the upper limit of the gluteus maximus and the lower internal area are both defined. Once the posterior zones are completed, liposuction of the inner thigh is completed with the patient in the supine position.[15,16] In contrast, we prefer 3-mm Mercedes cannulas for deep Lipoplasty in females. This is because we need soft transitions between the lower back (green zone) and the upper gluteal region (red zone) in addition to a soft blending towards the trochanteric depression. This area is difficult to access from the central intergluteal incision; so special cannulas are designed for this purpose (40 cm-long and 3-mm curved Mercedes cannula). Lipoaspiration of the lower and lateral gluteal areas is done through the infragluteal incisions. The inner thigh must be carefully sculpted to avoid abrupt transitions from the mid-inner tight adhesion area. On the lateral lower gluteal area, a negative space is created to blend the deep extraction in the lateral thigh and the gluteus to create a rounded shape.[17]

Regarding superficial liposuction, in men we aim for a sharp definition of the area above the gluteus maximus and at the lumbar rhomboid surroundings, including the erector spinae muscles. The gluteus medius will require fat grafting to enhance the butterfly appearance of the buttock and its squared shape. Comparatively, in women the superficial lipoplasty will depend on the degree of definition and how masculine they want their buttocks. In general, we advocate for soft transitions between muscle borders and aim to achieve a round shaped buttock. We also carve the rhombus of Michaelis and erector spinae muscles to improve the volumetric perception of the buttock; however, we do not recommend fat grafting of such muscles as it is not necessary (**Fig. 7**).

Carving the negative spaces allow transitions between concavities and convexities over the upper border of the gluteus maximus, the trochanteric depression, and the medial infra-gluteal fold. These areas should be defined more sharply in men compared to women, however, remember that there is an in-between definition for both depending on gender identification and individual preferences. Thorough liposuction is done over the lower flank areas to overlap its definition with the upper portion of the gluteus medius (intergluteal crease access). A sharp edge must be also created in the anterior zone over the tensor fascia latae muscle, then we do a transition zone moving posteriorly towards the gluteus maximus

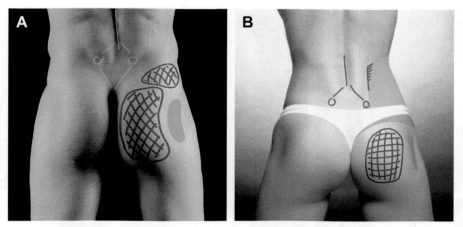

Fig. 10. The masculine buttock requires a butterfly shape (*A*) and a sharp definition of the gluteus medius with intramuscular fat grafting. The gender-neutral buttock (*B*) has features from both, then it can be the result of either the masculinization of a female's buttock or the feminization of a male's buttock. In effect, trochanteric depression is no longer a deep space but rather a linear definition (*B*). The green and red zones have to be considered and the gluteus medius is usually not grafted.

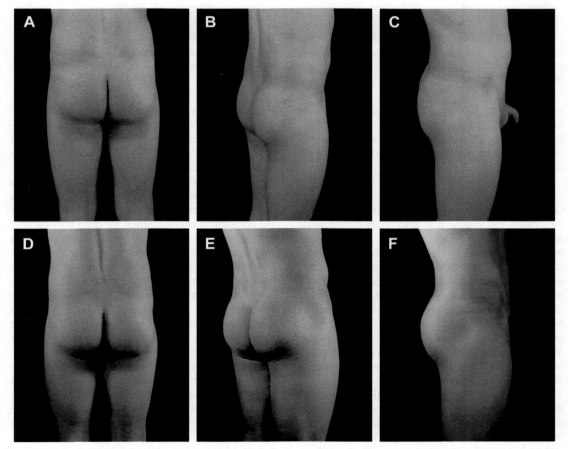

Fig. 11. Male patient who underwent the dynamic definition of the gluteal area including the posterior torso (*A–C*). Look how the buttock shape has been enhanced towards an athletic and squared shape (*D–F*).

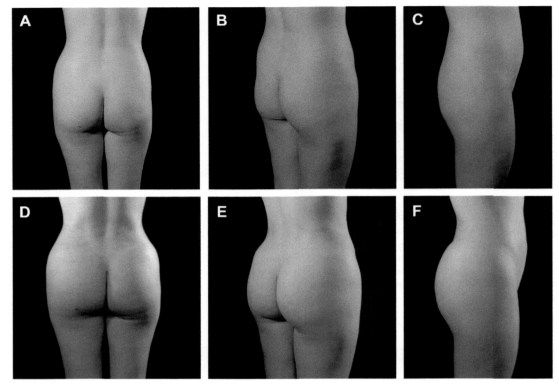

Fig. 12. Female patient undergoing the dynamic definition of the gluteal area and the lower limbs (*A–C*). Postoperative photographs (*D–F*) show a rounder buttock with the slim definition of the waist and the legs forming a continuum soft silhouette.

and superiorly reaching the gluteus medius. A curved cannula can be used for this purpose. Each zone is carefully revised, and refinements can be done depending on individual situations (**Fig. 8**).

Holometric fat grafting
One of the latest improvements in buttocks surgery has been the safety but also multi-dimensional approach of buttocks adipose tissue transfer.[2,13,18–20] In certain states (ie, Florida), it is now mandatory to use real-time intraoperative ultrasound while attempting buttock lipoinjection.[13,18,21–23] The surgeon must ensure the proper plane for which the graft will be placed and the distribution of the graft after injection. A proper mapping before lipoinjection including a blood vessel assessment through doppler mode are safe practices to get used to in order to decrease complications and improve the aesthetic outcomes.

Our technique for fat grafting (FG) has been improved along with our continuing expertise in body contouring. It is based on the current concepts about Static Injection, Migration and Equalization but modified to harmonize with the patient individual preferences and gender Identification.[24]

Multiple cadaveric studies have shown the peculiar anatomic structure of the gluteal area, specifically about compartments, deep fascia and superficial fascia.[6,18,22,25] These compartments allow the surgeon to place different amounts of adipose grafts in different locations so as to provide an individualized shape of the glutes (**Figs. 9** and **10**). Although different approaches are used for FG consistent with evidence for graft survival and safety,[18,26] we use 3- or 4-mm blunt cannulas attached to 60 mL syringes (manual mode) for Intramuscular FG of the gluteus medius and subcutaneous lipoinjection of the trochanteric depression. We couple a 4-mm basket cannula to MicroAire and use a peristaltic pump device (EVL–Expansion Vibration Lipofilling) to perform static injection at the subcutaneous layer. The proximal attachment is connected to a sterile bottle trap in which the adipose graft is ready for reinjection. Decantation is used to isolate viable fat cells from saline and blood cell components. The remaining supernatant is processed and prepared for fat grafting. The gluteal pillars must be grafted in patients who suffer infragluteal fold ptosis and/ or lack of projection of the posterior thigh. However, do not over-graft the whole zone as residual

251

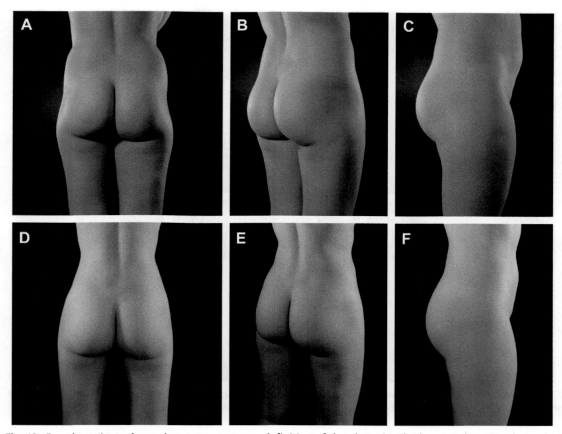

Fig. 13. Female patient who underwent an extreme definition of the glutes (*A–C*). The postoperative photos (*D–F*) show a defined and athletic shape of her buttocks, but still feminine.

bulking may appear. Deep strokes should be avoided, instead use a single injection and then equalization. There is no need to graft the trochanteric depression in round and "A"-shaped buttocks, but it is mandatory for square, and "V"-shaped. The grafting of this area should start from the top to the bottom with small volumes and through continuous strokes. Symmetry must be evaluated through photographs and multi-angle visualization inside the OR. Once the posterior zone is finished, some additional definitions can be done in the anterior zone (thigh and flank). Finally, we place a drain (Blake drain–Johnson®) at the subcutaneous space through the intergluteal crease incision to allow residual fluid drainage. Incisions are closed using a continuous subdermal stitching to avoid the graft leakage. High-absorbent pads are placed over the incisions, followed by the application of a garment and foam vest to facilitate skin adhesion.

Post-operative procedures

Patients requiring >5000 mL of fat extraction, as well as those requiring additional procedures or having comorbidities, such as hypertension or diabetes, should be admitted for overnight observation. Garments and foam vests should be used for 8-12 weeks (**Figs. 11–14**). We use only mild compression for those zones who were subject to fat grafting. Therapeutic lymphatic massage is recommended 2 days before surgery to activate lymphatics towards the inguinal lymph nodes on the inner thigh and daily sessions 10 to 20 times after surgery. Patients may perform isometric workouts to the lower limbs and glutes only 8 weeks after surgery. They might engage in stretching exercises the very next day after surgery. Drains should be assessed at each appointment with the therapist and should be removed on postoperative days 3 to 7 once drainage is less than 50 cc per 24 hours. Although the supine position is recommended during resting, there is no strict contra-indication on positioning. Early mobilization is promoted.

Complications

Although gluteal augmentation via autologous fat grafting techniques has been associated with a

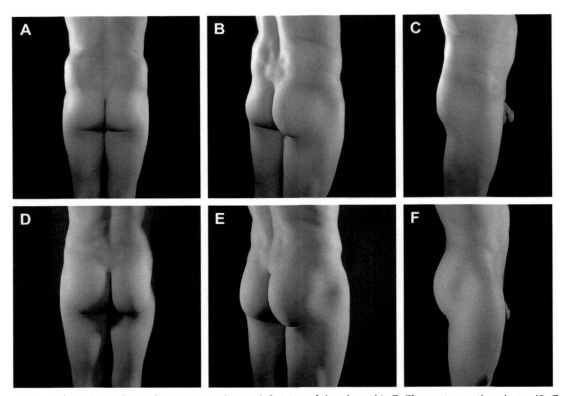

Fig. 14. Male patient who underwent a moderate definition of the glutes (A–C). The postoperative photos (D–F) show a round projected buttock, but still with the squared masculine shape.

lower complication rate when compared with implants (10.5% vs 30.5%, respectively), series of patients have documented complications including contour irregularities, fat necrosis, seroma, infection, oil cysts, hematoma, paresthesia, postsurgical pain as an intermittent burning sensation in the flank, fat embolism, pulmonary embolism, deep venous thromboembolism, and death.[27–29] According to the statistics of the International Society of Aesthetic Plastic Surgery, the estimated mortality rate of gluteal fat augmentation was one in 20,117 cases, and the estimated rate of nonfatal fat embolism was one in 9,530 cases.[28] The use of autologous tissues avoids the complications associated with gluteal implants, which include seroma, capsular contracture, implant migration, wound-healing issues, thinning of native tissues, implant palpability, and implant-related infections and exposures.[29] However, the plane of adipose graft injection can increase the risk of developing fatal outcomes. The risk of death is 16 times greater when fat graft is performed intramuscularly.[28] Multiple theories address this issue, one of them being the "direct hit" theory, in which due to direct trauma of the nearby blood vessels, fat is injected into the bloodstream.[30] Nonetheless, some of the surgeons who

documented fat emboli complications affirm not using the intramuscular plane for fat injection, and this lead to the proposal of the phenomenon of deep intramuscular migration, by which the fat injected in the intramuscular plane under certain pressure is forced to follow the least resistance path towards the deeper planes, causing traction induced venous tears which may lead to passive fat embolization.[30] Surgeons must always take the necessary precautions to avoid any additional risks when performing fat grafting; in addition to those from the gluteal task force,[13,21] we recommend large and single-holed cannulas for the IM gluteus medius procedure, always set the cannula perpendicular to the pedicle, place the graft in the medial muscular zone, place the tip of the cannula far from the main vascular pedicle and avoid multiple injections. There are all protective measures against pulmonary fat emboli because they reduce the risk of injury to vessels, and they are less likely to bend following and undesired path.[31]

SUMMARY

Differences in gluteal reshaping are no longer gender-based but actually will depend on each individual preference. Although gender premises for dynamic definition liposculpture still apply, the in-between features for both male and female pa-tients allow the surgeon to perform a broader spectrum of procedures that can be individualized according to muscular structure, desires and gender ID. Gluteus medius and gluteus maximus adipose grafts improve the volumetric appearance of the glutes, though a detailed technique is required to avoid complications and improve the outcomes. Unless requested by the patient, do not fat Graft the trochanteric depression in men, this will result in a feminizing facet (round gluteus).

CLINICS CARE POINTS

- Anatomy is the cornerstone for dynamic definition liposculpture.
- Do NOT perform exhaustive superficial liposuction over the adhesion zones of the glutes nor the thighs.
- Avoid over-resection of the gluteal red zone. It will be very hard to correct afterwards.
- Sharp edges and muscular definition are suitable for all male and only female with extreme definition.
- Round glutes and soft definition are for most female and males who want a more feminine appearance.
- Real-time ultrasound imaging is compulsory for any Fat grafting attempt to the buttocks.
- Intramuscular fat grafting is only suitable for the gluteus medius (regarding the buttock area).
- Dynamic definition liposculpture requires a steady learning curve and detailed anatomic concepts to successfully achieve the volumetric perception of the gluteal area and its definition in different degrees of muscularization.

DISCLOSURE

The authors did not have financial interest nor receive any financial support of the products or devices mentioned in this article. All other authors declare that they have no conflicts of interest.

FUNDING

The authors received no financial support for the research, authorship, and publication of this article.

REFERENCES

1. Centeno RF, Sood A, Young VL. Clinical anatomy in aesthetic gluteal contouring. Clin Plast Surg 2018; 45(2):145–57. Available at: https://pubmed.ncbi.nlm.nih.gov/29519484/.
2. Che D-H, Xiao Z-B. Gluteal augmentation with fat grafting: literature review. Aesthetic Plast Surg 2021; 45(4):1633–41. Available at: https://pubmed.ncbi.nlm.nih.gov/33216176/.
3. Roberts TL, Weinfeld AB, Bruner TW, et al. "Universal" and ethnic ideals of beautiful buttocks are best obtained by autologous micro fat grafting and liposuction. Clin Plast Surg 2006;33(3):371–94. Available at: https://pubmed.ncbi.nlm.nih.gov/16818095/.
4. Cuenca-Guerra R, Quezada J. What makes buttocks beautiful? A review and classification of the determinants of gluteal beauty and the surgical techniques to achieve them. Aesthetic Plast Surg 2004;28(5):340–7. https://pubmed.ncbi.nlm.nih.gov/15666052/.
5. Mendieta CG. Classification system for gluteal evaluation. Clin Plast Surg 2006;33(3):333–46. Available at: https://pubmed.ncbi.nlm.nih.gov/16818092/.
6. Si L., Li Z., Fu L., et al., Gluteal Fold: Cadaveric Dissection of the Superficial Fascial System in the Buttock and Anatomy-based Gluteal Liposculpture [published online ahead of print, 2023 May 22]. Plast Reconstr Surg. 2023;10.1097/PRS.0000000000010723. https://doi.org/10.1097/PRS.0000000000010723.
7. Hoyos A. Gluteal region. In: Perez M, editor. Total definer: atlas of body sculpting. 1st ed. New York: Thieme; 2023. p. 289–327.
8. Illouz Y. The fat cell "graft": a new technique to fill depressions. Plast Reconstr Surg 1986;78:122–3.
9. Mladick R. Combined gluteoplasty: liposuction and lipoinjection discussion. Plast Reconstr Surg 1999; 104:1532–3.
10. Cao W, Sheng L. Buttock augmentation with fat grafting. Clin Plast Surg 2023;50(1):171–9.
11. Aslani A, Del Vecchio DA. Composite buttock augmentation: the next frontier in gluteal aesthetic surgery. Plast Reconstr Surg 2019;144(6):1312–21.
12. Senderoff DM. Aesthetic surgery of the buttocks using implants: practice-based recommendations. Aesthetic Surg J 2016;36(5):559–76.
13. Del Vecchio D, Kenkel JM. Practice advisory on gluteal fat grafting. Aesthetic Surg J 2022;42(9): 1019–29. Available at: https://pubmed.ncbi.nlm.nih.gov/35404456/.
14. Hoyos AE, Perez ME, Domínguez-Millán R. Male aesthetics for the gluteal area: anatomy and algorithm for surgical approach for dynamic definition body contouring. Plast Reconstr Surg 2020;146(2): 284–93.

15. Cárdenas-Camarena L, Trujillo-Méndez R, Díaz-Barriga JC. Tridimensional combined gluteoplasty: liposuction, buttock implants, and fat transfer. Plast Reconstr Surg 2020;146(1):53–63. Available at: https://pubmed.ncbi.nlm.nih.gov/32590643/.

16. Hoyos A. Lower limb. In: Perez M, editor. Total definer: atlas of body sculpting. 1st ed. New York: Thieme; 2023. p. 328–75.

17. Mendieta C, Stuzin JM. Gluteal augmentation and enhancement of the female silhouette: analysis and technique. Plast Reconstr Surg 2018;141(2):306–11. https://pubmed.ncbi.nlm.nih.gov/29369983/.

18. Del Vecchio DA, Villanueva NL, Mohan R, et al. Clinical implications of gluteal fat graft migration: a dynamic anatomical study. Plast Reconstr Surg 2018;142(5):1180–92. Available at. https://pubmed.ncbi.nlm.nih.gov/30102666/.

19. Toledo LS. Gluteal augmentation with fat grafting. Clin Plast Surg 2015;42(2):253–61.

20. Condé-Green A, Kotamarti V, Nini KT, et al. Fat grafting for gluteal augmentation. Plast Reconstr Surg 2016;138(3). 437e–46e.

21. Villanueva NL, Del Vecchio DA, Afrooz PN, et al. Staying safe during gluteal fat transplantation. Plast Reconstr Surg 2018;141(1):79–86.

22.. Frojo G, Halani SH, Pessa JE, et al. Deep subcutaneous gluteal fat compartments: anatomy and clinical implications. Aesthetic Surg J 2023;43(1):76–83.

23. Del Vecchio DA, Wall SJ, Mendieta CG, et al. Safety comparison of abdominoplasty and brazilian butt lift: what the literature tells us. Plast Reconstr Surg 2021; 148(6):1270–7.

24. Pazmiño P, Del Vecchio D. Static Injection, Migration, and Equalization (SIME): A New Paradigm for Better. Aesthet Surg J 2023;sjad142. https://doi.org/10.1093/asj/sjad142.

25. Pirri C, Fede C, Petrelli L, et al. An anatomical comparison of the fasciae of the thigh: a macroscopic, microscopic and ultrasound imaging study. J Anat 2021;238(4):999–1009.

26. Del Vecchio D, Wall S. Expansion vibration lipofilling: a new technique in large-volume fat transplantation. Plast Reconstr Surg 2018;141(5). 639e–49e. Available at: https://pubmed.ncbi.nlm.nih.gov/29465484/.

27. Abboud MH, Dibo SA, Abboud NM. Power-assisted liposuction and lipofilling: techniques and experience in large-volume fat grafting. Aesthetic Surg J 2020;40(2):180–90. Available at: https://academic.oup.com/asj/article/40/2/180/5306364.

28. Cansancao AL, Condé-Green A, Gouvea Rosique R, et al. "Brazilian butt lift" performed by board-certified brazilian plastic surgeons: reports of an expert opinion survey. Plast Reconstr Surg 2019; 144(3):601–9. Available at: https://pubmed.ncbi.nlm.nih.gov/31461012/.

29. Ordenana C, Dallapozza E, Said S, et al. Objectifying the risk of vascular complications in gluteal augmentation with fat grafting: a latex casted cadaveric study. Aesthetic Surg J 2020;40(4):402–9. Available at: https://pubmed.ncbi.nlm.nih.gov/31665218/.

30. O'Neill RC, Abu-Ghname A, Davis MJ, et al. Fat grafting in plastic surgery: the role of fat grafting in buttock augmentation. Semin Plast Surg 2020; 34(1):38. Available at:/pmc/articles/PMC7023974/.

31. Mofid MM, Teitelbaum S, Suissa D, et al. Report on mortality from gluteal fat grafting: recommendations from the ASERF task force. Aesthetic Surg J 2017; 37(7):796–806. Available at: https://pubmed.ncbi.nlm.nih.gov/28369293/.

The S-Curve®
Clinical Importance of the Gluteal Ligaments in Efficacious Fat Transfer

Ashkan Ghavami, MD[a,b,*], Neil M. Vranis, MD[b]

KEYWORDS

- S-Curve® • Subcutaneous gluteal lipoaugmentation • Gluteal anatomy
- Gluteal subcutaneous ligaments • Brazilian butt lift safety • Gluteal fat transfer • Buttock fat transfer

KEY POINTS

- Previous anatomic studies confirm the consistent presence of predictable location of dermofascial attachments in the gluteal region.
- Optimizing aesthetic outcomes while maintaining safety requires detailed anatomic knowledge of the internal subcutaneous structural landscape, including large named ligaments and areas of dense fibrous banding, which influence the overall buttock shape and structure.
- Real-time tactile feedback with each excursion of the cannula permits the surgeon to detect and precisely release internal ligamentous structures creating a space for lipoexpansion while minimizing the risk of contour irregularities and "blowouts." In addition, completing the fat transfer using a hybrid technique[1] with power-assisted direct "manual" canula injection provides improved predictability without compromise of safety.

INTRODUCTION

Safety in gluteal augmentation has recently garnered significant attention among plastic surgeons, patients, and the media. A multisociety task force was commissioned to review this specific procedure as an effort to minimize the morbidity and mortality that has been directly linked to fat embolism and death. A thorough understanding of regional anatomy and ensuring that the cannula remains in the subcutaneous space during fat transfer were the two main recommendations.[2] The possibility of dynamic fat migration from the subcutaneous fat compartment to the deep muscular compartment once the gluteal fascia has been pierced[3,4] has led to a paradigm shift from intramuscular to subcutaneous-only fat grafting.[5] This trend magnifies the importance of understanding relevant subcutaneous ligamentous anatomy and their influence on buttock shape/support.

Liposuction coupled with fat transfer for autologous gluteal augmentation demands artistic vision and technical skill to sculpt aesthetically pleasing concave and convex curves with gentle, harmonious transitions from the upper back down to the midthigh. Augmenting the buttock while maintaining naturally appearing proportions and respecting the necessary structural pillars to maintain gluteal shape longevity remains a challenging endeavor. The ideal aesthetically pleasing "S-shaped" gluteal silhouette constructed by the S-Curve® procedure has been previously described.[6] In addition to shape outline, the "S" also stands for "safety" and "subcutaneous," reminding surgeons that safety should never be compromised. This article provides clinical insights along with technical considerations involved in judicious gluteal ligamentous release allowing for precise augmentation, delicate curves, yet adequate preservation of underlying

[a] Division of Plastic and Reconstructive Surgery, Department of Surgery, David Geffen School of Medicine at UCLA, Los Angeles, CA, USA; [b] Private Practice, Ghavami Plastic Surgery, 433 North Camden Drive, Suite 780, Beverly Hills, CA 90210, USA
* Corresponding author. 433 North Camden Drive, Suite 780, Beverly Hills, CA 90210.
E-mail address: ashghavami@yahoo.com

Clin Plastic Surg 50 (2023) 553–561
https://doi.org/10.1016/j.cps.2023.06.001

critical structures to prevent contour deformities and downstream complications.

ANATOMIC CONSIDERATIONS

A thorough understanding of subcutaneous structural anatomy and more importantly, how the ligaments collectively dictate external contours, is critical when performing the S-Curve® procedure (**Fig. 1**). Multiple cadaver dissection studies have been performed to evaluate the anatomic location, consistency, and implications of the gluteal ligaments.

Two important fascial adhesions mark the medial and inferior borders of each buttock. The gluteal cleft adhesion is vertically oriented near the midline, separating the two buttocks; whereas, the transverse gluteal crease adhesion separates the buttock from the posterior thigh. The latter is also referred to as the inferior gluteal crease. Both of these adhesions originate from the gluteal fascial and insert onto the dermis. The sacrocutaneous ligament originates superomedially from the lateral margin of the sacrum and extends in a curvilinear fashion laterally to interdigitate with the dermis

and other less dense adhesions tethered to the posterior iliac crest.[7] The lateral aspect of the ligament becomes narrowed and less taut. The broad, fan-shaped ischiocutaneous ligament originates from the inferomedial corner of each buttock. This is at the confluence of the ischial tuberosity, the gluteal cleft, and gluteal crease adhesions, and fans outward at an oblique superolateral trajectory. It was found to be the most dense and difficult to pierce with a cannula ex vivo.[7] This broad ligament offers a potential evolutionary benefit because it covers and protects the deep neurovascular structures, important to lower extremity viability. Clinically, certain patients with a pronounced ischiocutaneous ligament present with a diagonal area of flattening in the inferomedial quadrant of the buttock (**Fig. 2**). In severe cases, this is flanked by areas that are significantly less tethered thereby creating a "double-bubble" appearance. Appreciating this finding on physical examination is predictive that adequate release of the ischiocutaneous ligament and creating meaningful expansion in this quadrant is challenging.

A separate, more recent, cadaveric study identified seven fat compartments in the deep subcu-

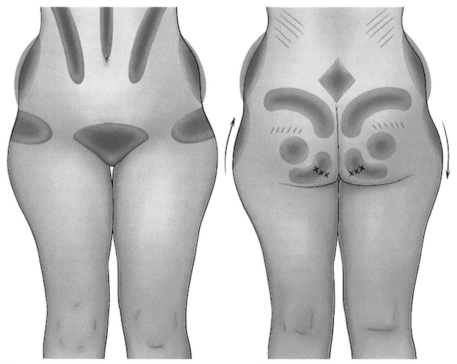

Fig. 1. An illustration that demonstrates the pre-operative planning/considerations in performing liposuction and gluteal augmentation via fat transfer. Red highlights the areas of reduction, while the green depicts which parts of the buttock will be infiltrated with fat. The arrows depict pelvic tilt and the 'xxx' are areas that will require extensive release due to strong osseocutaneous ligamentous attachment.

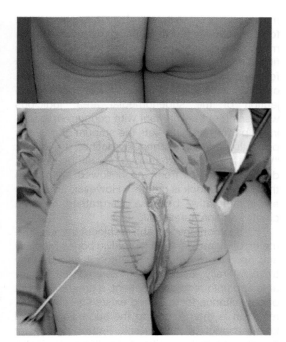

Fig. 2. Preoperative posterior view photographs of the buttocks, exemplifying the transcutaneous visibility of a prominent ischiocutaneous ligament (*top*). This finding is observed as an oblique linear area of flattening that is found in the inferomedial quadrant of the buttock. Intraoperative release of the ligament with a 4-mm basket cannula (*bottom*) allows for adequate inferomedial expansion and treatment of congenital contour abnormalities caused by the ischiocutaneous ligament.

taneous fat layer.[8] The superficial gluteal fascia system, analogous to Scarpa fascia in the abdomen, is readily visualized on ultrasound and separates the superficial and deep compartments of the subcutaneous space. Using multiple static injections to simulate static lipofilling procedures, the authors found that the dyed fat spreads within each compartment but does not permeate the boundaries, the superficial fascia system, or the gluteus maximus fascia.[8] They identified three medial compartments (superior, middle, and inferior), a central compartment, and three lateral compartments (superior, middle, inferior). The findings also correlated with their intraoperative experience and observation that increased resistance of the cannula was consistently encountered along the trajectory of these internal retaining ligaments. This phenomenon aligns with multiple other reports in the literature. Pazmino and Del Vecchio had previously described the concept of static injection, migration, and equalization (SIME) for gluteal augmentation.[9] For each compartment filled, they note that there is a discrete area of augmentation affirming the presence of internal dermofascial

retaining ligaments that do not allow fat to readily permeate.[10] Lastly, the anatomic consistency is in accordance with descriptions by multiple authors. For example, the ischiocutaneous ligament first described by Ghavami and coworkers[7] runs between the compartments Frojo and colleagues[8] labeled as middle and inferior along the medial aspect of each buttock, further corroborating their findings.

SURGICAL TECHNIQUE
S-Curve® Incision and Access Points

Typically, the S-Curve® procedure is successfully performed through two posterior port incisions (one on each side). These are made on the superior aspect of the buttock along the gluteal-flank junction, allowing the surgeon adequate degrees of freedom to perform liposuction of the back, flank, and lateral thighs. The same access site is subsequently used for lipofilling and buttock reshaping. A caveat is when two additional (one on each side) port incisions are made along the inferior gluteal crease. In the senior author's practice this is required in approximately 60% of cases. The indications for these additional access sites are:

1. Medial thigh adiposity extends posteriorly and requires liposuction from an anterior and posterior trajectory. This allows for better cross-tunneling and decreases the risk of contour irregularities. The patient's body habitus may also prevent the surgeon from accessing the entire fat compartment solely from an anterior access site.
2. Preoperative assessment of the gluteal quadrant reveals an extremely flat inferomedial quadrant. This is a consequence of a stout ischiocutaneous ligament. A strong ligament requires biplanar release from two separate access points.
3. Intraoperatively the surgeon encounters a very tight ischiocutaneous ligament (similar concept as above) that prevents adequate expansion after release by an exploding tip cannula from the superior to inferior direction. The additional inferior gluteal crease incision allows for cross-tunneling and thus a more extensive ligamentous release.
4. Preoperative presence of "banana-roll" deformity. An inferior gluteal crease incision allows for close proximity to treat this deformity. Conservative liposuction and fat grafting can be precisely performed minimizing the risk of exacerbating the "banana roll" appearance.

One philosophy is that separate access sites should be used for liposuction and lipofilling. The principal argument is that the numerous passes from large-bore (greater than 4 mm) basket cannulas create an expansive subcutaneous potential space. When fat is transferred through the same port sites, albeit in an adjacent territory, there is a theoretic risk for the fat to displace retrograde through the injection tunnels and into the potential space that was created during the liposuction portion of the case. Pressure differentials may encourage retrograde fat migration because the gluteal area is under high pressure given that it has been filled with intension to generate expansion, whereas the flank, sacrum, and back that have been thoroughly debulked thereby creating a low-pressure system. The senior author has performed more than 3000 S-Curve® gluteal fat transfers since 2008, using the same access site for liposuction and lipofilling. Repeat preparation of the back with betadine between the two segments of the operation minimizes contamination and the risk for infection. Also, a meticulous water-tight closure of the port sites seals the internal system preventing any egress of the fat. By following these tenents, the senior author has not observed any clinically relevant issues with fat displacement or contour irregularities between the time of surgery and any subsequent follow-up visits (short-term and long-term).

Sequence of Operation

During the preoperative consultation, areas of liposuction for fat harvest are customized based on the location of excess adiposity. Delicate suggestions can be made while respecting patient desires. With the patient in the supine position, adherence to the widely accepted liposuction principles of separation, aspiration, and fat equalization (SAFE)[10] enables the surgeon to harvest fat while sculpting the abdomen, flanks, and inner thighs. In patients with hip dips that extend anteriorly, a modest amount of fat transfer is performed to fill the anterior deficit from the supine position.

Once the patient is safely turned to the prone position, SAFE liposuction techniques finalize flank contours, sculpt an aesthetically pleasing diamond-shaped sacrum, and enhance back/arm definition. Surgeons should remain mindful that the purpose of liposuction is not only to harvest fat, but also plays a critical role in the reshaping of the entire torso silhouette. It establishes a smooth S-Curve® transition between the lower back and upper buttock poles and the flanks/waistline and lateral buttock and outer thigh/hip region.

Gluteal ligaments are considerably more adherent medially and become more flaccid as

they continue laterally, an observation consistent for the superior and inferior ligamentous attachments. The superiomedial aspect of the buttock is filled first. The sacrocutaneous ligament accounts for the depth and structure of the intergluteal sulcus.[11] Therefore, to manipulate the shape and projection of the superiomedial area, judicious weakening of the ligament with concurrent lipofilling is performed. This sets the amount of superior projection and simultaneously defines the inferior "V" of the diamond-shaped sacral borders. A defined transition from the hollowed sacrum to the upper buttock is created. However, an artistic eye is imperative, because overgrafting this area creates an unnatural shelf.

The sacrocutaneous and ischiocutaneous ligaments originate deep on the pelvic bones medially and become more superficial and flaccid as they travel laterally. Because the lateral extent is variable and unique to each patient, a greater amount of capacitance for lipofilling exists laterally. Thus, attention is then turned to the superolateral and lateral aspect of the buttock. Feathering the fat creates a smooth transition to the flanks. Typically, a small degree of widening is needed to match the width of the lateral thigh, set by the intertrochanteric distance. An additional consideration is the width of waist that has been altered by reshaping of the flanks. Crowdsourcing studies have validated that the golden ratio of 1:1.6 is the "ideal," aesthetically pleasing waist/hip ratio.[12]

Continuing with the top-down approach, fat transferred to the center of the buttock and midlateral adds volume and projection. Mendieta[13] has previously described this area as the C-point. Care is taken to prevent overwidening the buttock. Preinjection with tumescent solution is helpful to pre-expand this region, which then more easily accommodates fat. This area is typically very adherent with a complex interface between the superficial and deep fascial planes making it a challenge to achieve optimal volume expansion. This is followed by transferring fat to the inferomedial section, which is also a challenging area to expand given the confluence of three ligamentous attachments. The ischiocutaneous ligament is the strongest and most important ligament to release. Meticulous, incremental release of the internal structures balances the capacity for expansion while maintaining enough support to prevent postoperative ptosis. Typically, the inferolateral aspect of the buttock does not require much fat, if at all. The final maneuver involves equalization of the fat grafts by internal cannula ligamentous releasing and/or external manual massaging preventing microcontour irregularities. In most cases, the senior author judiciously uses a syringe connected to a power-assisted cannula (hybrid technique[1]) to fine tune the shape in certain areas and equalize the distribution of injected fat. This maneuver is applied for the final 20% to 30% of the fat transferred. It is particularly useful in patients with prominent lateral gluteal depressions ("hip dips"), tight adherence of overlying buttock skin (athletic women with a thin subcutaneous layer), and those with an overall larger buttock.

The key to achieving an aesthetically pleasing S-Curve® result stems from the surgeon's ability to appreciate and create gentle transitions from areas of convexity to concavity. Removal of adiposity from areas of excess and transferring volume to areas that require augmentation, this procedure results in a complete, circumferential reshaping of the female silhouette. Abrupt transition points appear unnatural, are less aesthetically appealing, and should be avoided. Often times, one can appreciate two inflection points above the buttock on the far side of the posterior oblique view preoperatively. One is at the junction of upper back to superior flank and the second exists at the flank-buttock transition. After the S-Curve® procedure a gentle "S" curve, which begins at the level of the upper back and continues down to the midthigh, is appreciated in the posterior, three-quarter, and anterior views (Fig. 3). This implies that there is only a single convex to concave inflection point above the buttock and one below. Intermittently, throughout the procedure, the surgeon is encouraged to assess the symmetry, size, shape, and relative proportions from all sides of the operating room table to make incremental changes as their artistic eye deems necessary.

Several prominent surgeons who perform a large number of gluteal fat transfer operations comment on the significance of tactile feedback regarding resistance experienced with each pass of the cannula. This enables the surgeon to appreciate the presence and strength of internal structures in various areas of the buttocks. With each pistoning motion, the integrity of the internal structure loosens to a small degree. Using a flared Mercedes cannula or pickle fork with forceful swiping side-to-side motions (ie, deep aponeurotomy) can more aggressively release these internal ligaments. A focal loss of resistance alerts the surgeon that a complete release was performed. Caution must be applied to avoid overrelease with a complete loss of resistance over a broad area.

DISCUSSION

Familiarity with the internal gluteal fascial boundaries, fascial-dermal ligaments, and overall subcutaneous architecture allows the surgeon to properly evaluate and manipulate various structures to create an aesthetically pleasing buttock augmentation. The gluteal fascia acts as a fat-impermeable divider between superficial and deep planes protecting the muscles, sciatic nerve, and gluteal vessels.[4] Currently, ongoing investigations are evaluating the safety of subfascial and intramuscular fat injections. However, the most recent society task force composed of pioneers of gluteal augmentation universally advocate for certain safety precautions. The most important recommendation is to remain in the subcutaneous space, mitigating the risk of fat embolus and nerve injury.[4,7]

A critical fascial layer to consider is the deep gluteal fascia, which is a strong fascial layer, impermeable to fat graft migration unless its integrity is damaged or punctured. Multiple cadaveric fat injection simulation studies have confirmed the integrity of the deep gluteal fascia, which separates the subcutaneous fat from the muscles, nerves, and important vasculature.[4,8] The deep gluteal fascia also acts as the foundation or origin for many fasciocutaneous ligaments. The large, named ligaments include the gluteal cleft adhesion and the transverse gluteal crease adhesion. The existence and consistence of other fasciocutaneous ligaments is evidenced by the seven compartments described by Frojo and colleagues.[8] These partitions between compartments fall under the umbrella term referred to as the subcutaneous structural architecture. This includes all of the oblique and perpendicular fibrous bands that associate the deep fascia, superficial fascia, and dermis. These bands are also the anatomic basis of cellulite.[14] In addition to the named and unnamed fasciocutaneous adhesions, two stout osseocutaneous ligaments exist: the ischiocutaneous and sacrocutaneous ligaments.

Collectively, the osseocutaneous and fasciocutaneous ligaments provide structural integrity and shape to the buttock. The buttock projects beyond its foundation, the thighs, in the standing position acting as a cantilever. This architectural concept suggests that the pelvic bones and gluteal fascia transverse ligaments must retain enough strength to support the buttock's weight against a vertically oriented gravitational force. Inevitably, inadequate structural integrity leads to downward descent and buttock ptosis.

Compliance and capacitance are additional physics concepts that should be considered during this procedure. In a prospective study by Cansancao and colleagues,[5] the 1-year fat retention rate exceeded 80% after an average injection volume of 520 mL per buttock (range, 420–600 mL), when the fat was placed in the subcutaneous

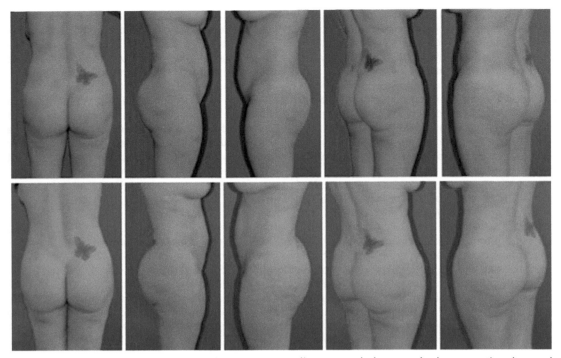

Fig. 3. Preoperative (*top row*) and 13 months postoperative (*bottom row*) photographs demonstrating the gentle S-shaped outline from the back to the midthigh region after an S-Curve® procedure as seen from the posterior view (*left column*). The fat redistribution from the flanks to the buttock augments the projection in lateral view (*middle two columns*) and produces gentle transitions between areas of convexity and concavity in the posterior oblique view (*right two columns*). One can appreciate two inflection points (back-to-flank and flank-to-buttock) on the far side of the body in the preoperative posterior oblique view, whereas there is only a single concave-to-convex transition point in the postoperative posterior oblique photograph.

space. In addition to confirming the reliability of high-volume fat transfer, this study demonstrates a significant amount of capacitance that can be created in the gluteal subcutaneous space with appropriate release of the underlying structures. Compliance is a property directly correlated to the degree of soft tissue laxity determined by the degree of skin laxity and overall adherence of the dermis to the underlying fascia by way of the subcutaneous ligaments. Capacitance is the amount of additional volume that a system can tolerate. These two variables are related but not interchangeable. Skin laxity is manipulated with radiofrequency and thermal-based treatments designed to tighten dermal collagen; however, this is outside the scope of this article. Youthful patients with minimal skin laxity tend to have a far superior postoperative appearance after fat transfer despite the less compliance and capacitance of their soft tissues. Conversely, patients with excessive soft tissue laxity and thus too much compliance, are not candidates for fat transfer gluteal augmentation procedures; instead, resective

procedures are warranted. This illustrates that simply increasing capacitance is not always the appropriate solution.

The S-Curve® procedure, developed by the senior author, relies on attentive preoperative observation, incremental ligamentous release, receptive real-time tactile feedback, and meticulous fat transfer techniques. As described previously, after fat has been harvested and processed, the initial focus is on release and lipofilling the medial aspect of the buttock. In doing so, particular attention must be paid to angulation of the cannula because this is a danger zone for cannula misadventures to be deeper than expected and pierce the gluteal fascia putting the sciatic nerve and large blood vessels at risk. The ligaments discussed in this article traverse from deeper structures to the dermis, thus, release should occur while they traverse the subcutaneous space. The trajectory of the cannula must remain flat or even point upward while injecting fat and releasing the subcutaneous ligaments. A gluteal lipofilling simulation-cadaveric study performed in Mexico, demonstrated that a

45° downward trajectory–entry point at the lateral sacrum in a superior to inferior direction, puts the cannula tip in close proximity to the superior and inferior gluteal artery/vein. However, the tip remains intramuscularly with a 30° downward trajectory from the same entry point.[15] This cadaveric study was performed with flexion at the hip, "jackknife" position, simulating appropriate intraoperative conditions. One can extrapolate from these findings that even less acute cannula angulation is recommended to remain in the subcutaneous plane when injecting from the superior to inferior direction in the medial half of the buttock.

An additional implication of ligamentous rigidity includes cannula misguidance. As mentioned elsewhere in this issue, patient positioning along with cannula trajectory and angulation during fat transfer is critical to remain in the subcutaneous space and avoid disruption of the deeper structures. As the cannula passes through the stout ligaments, the torque may cause deflection of the cannula such that the tip is inadvertently directed deep and may penetrate the gluteus muscular fascia leading to unintentional large vessel injury.[6] To prevent cannula flexibility, many surgeons advocate for passing a stiff, power-assisted, vibrating liposuction cannula in a multidirectional and multilayered fashion before fat transfer to disrupt the fibrous matrix and allow for expansion (increases buttock capacitance).[16] Others, recommend using expansion vibration lipofilling with a roller-pump-propelled fat to improve efficiency by simultaneously disrupting the recipient stromal tissue, internally expanding and filling the space with fat grafts.[17] Descriptions of this technique involve using large-bore roller-pump tubing and cannulas to maximize efficiency and safely decrease operative times. A more recent evolution in technique championed by leaders in this field involves published SIME.[9] This technique minimizes the number of cannula passes during the fat grafting portion of the procedure allowing diffusion gradients and external massage/pressure to distribute the adipose grafts. Although the precision of graft placement is compromised, a benefit is that there is less disruption of the recipient architecture and structure by minimizing the number of passes and damage caused by the vibrating cannula. This also minimizes surgeon fatigue and the operative time spent injecting fat. Selective ligamentous release can then be performed subsequent to injection allowing for gluteal shaping.

Purists would argue that the bolus fat injection concept contradicts the Coleman philosophy of depositing fat grafts in small aliquots with each pass of the cannula to maximize graft to blood vessel proximity ensuring high levels of engraftment. Some argue that large-volume lipofilling is an entirely different operation with different physiology given the less-compliant buttock tissue compared with other, more compliant bodily areas, such as the aging deflated face. Replacing volume that previously existed is different than using the fat to expand and contour an area that was not convex in the first place.[17] Future studies are needed to assess the yield, granuloma formation, fat necrosis, and other outcomes with the SIME technique compared with traditional fat grafting methods.

Contrary to large-bolus injection techniques, repeated passes of the cannula before (prerelease) and during fat transfer interrupts the subcutaneous fibrous architecture and ligamentous structures, and thus, in effect merges these compartments. Certain technique articles advocate for the use of exploded-tip cannulas to release bands and diminish resistance in the tight areas, specifically the midlateral and inferolateral buttock. However, complete disruption of the gluteal ligaments or weakening the overall subcutaneous structural connective tissue by overzealous manipulation of the cannula can lead to a "blowout."[4,6] Clinically this is appreciated by loss of resistance on cannula excursion in a specific area. Fat injected migrates to this area following basic physics principles of pressure gradients, which has negative downstream effects, such as fat necrosis, seroma, and contour abnormalities.

Inferior buttock descent and ptosis are additional complications with a multifactorial cause. An excess or imbalance of fat transferred to the lower pole of the buttock coupled with excessive weakening of the inferior ligamentous support contribute to ptosis. Furthermore, effacement of the inferior gluteal crease adhesion blunts the transition from thigh to buttock, weakens the inferior support, and creates an unnatural-appearing transition. Ptosis can also be a downstream sequela of ligamentous overrelease that can present in the subacute recovery phase.[17] This should caution the novice surgeon to perform conservative, precise ligamentous releases allowing for expansion but not too much as to create structural instability.

SUMMARY

Reliably increasing the capacitance of the buttock to accommodate the fat transfer relies on manipulating the inherent tightness of the subcutaneous structural architecture. There is a certain amount of soft tissue elasticity throughout the buttock. The elasticity of ligaments is far less than the areas between the ligaments; thus, selective release

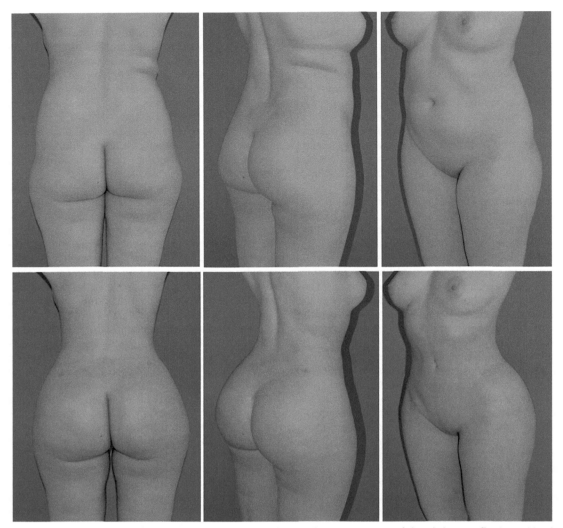

Fig. 4. This is a 30-year-old female desiring medium definition lipo-contouring of the abdomen, flanks and back. S-Curve® also includes precise fat transfer to the buttock for augmentation and re-shaping. Pre-operative photographs (top row) and 10 months post-operative (bottom row).

allows the tether points to release and prevent focal contour irregularities because of soft tissue tethering. This is done with a cannula, pitch-fork, or even power-assisted cannulas. However, the pretunneling technique, or power-assisted vibratory expansion lipofilling lacks precision and carries a high risk of overloosening the subcutaneous fibrous network. The novice surgeon should be wary that vibrations from the power-assisted handpieces blunts tactile feedback and may not appreciate the subtle differences in cannula resistance. It is encouraged to begin with a hand-held syringe and Toomey compatible cannulas such that a subtle change in resistance is appreciated with each pass.

The senior author has performed numerous S-Curve® procedures for more than two decades with excellent patient satisfaction, high levels of fat graft yield, and low complication rates. The syringe method allows for controlled and precise grafting that minimizes trauma to the adipocytes, unlike the theoretic crushing mechanism a roller pump may cause. A rigid cannula is preferred to avoid bending, which may cause misdirection and fat deposition deeper than intended. Additionally, the authors recommend extra caution when using expansion vibration devices (ie, power-assisted handpieces) coupled with aggressive cannulas (ie, large-bore basket cannulas) at the recipient site to minimize the risk of "blowout." Respecting the borders of the buttock formed by the fascial adhesions described previously maintains a natural aesthetic. Understanding the macrostructures and microstructures combined with careful and judicious release/weakening of the structural subcutaneous architecture allows for appropriate expansion and lipofilling while preventing flattening, contour irregularities, and "blowout" (**Fig. 4**).

CLINICS CARE POINTS

Pearls

- Precise, judicious, yet adequate release of gluteal ligaments allows for focal expansion, increased capacitance, and efficacious fat transfer with high recipient site survival rates.
- Real-time tactile feedback is imperative to appreciate the internal ligamentous landscape and degree of release performed with each pass of the cannula.
- Liposuction and lipofilling is safely performed through the same access site with minimal risk of unintended fat displacement.

Pitfalls

- Flattening and contour irregularities of the buttock is a consequence of attempted lipofilling with inadequate ligamentous release.
- Use of power-assisted vibratory hand pieces at the recipient site may blunt the subtle differences of resistance with each pass of the cannula, leading to unintended overrelease.
- Overzealous release of internal structural ligaments and bands can cause a "blowout" and/or contribute to postoperative buttock ptosis.

DISCLOSURE

Dr. A. Ghavami: Royalties from Thieme Pub, QMP and Consultant/Advisor for MTF Inc, Advisor/Marketing Partner InMode Inc.

REFERENCES

1. Ghavami A, Halani S, Amirlak B. The hybrid technique for autologous gluteal augmentation. Aesthetic Surg J 2023;5(2):1–6.
2. Del Vecchio D, Kenkel JM. Practice advisory on gluteal fat grafting. Aesthetic Surg J 2022;42(9):1019–29.
3. Del Vecchio DA, Villanueva NL, Mohan R, et al. Clinical implications of gluteal fat graft migration: a dynamic anatomical study. Plast Reconstr Surg 2018;142(5):1180–92.
4. Wall S, Delvecchio D, Teitelbaum S, et al. Subcutaneous migration: a dynamic anatomical study of gluteal fat grafting. Plast Reconstr Surg 2019;143(5):1343–51.
5. Cansancao AL, Conde-Green A, David JA, et al. Subcutaneous-only gluteal fat grafting: a prospective study of the long-term results with ultrasound analysis. Plast Reconstr Surg 2018;143(2):447–51.
6. Ghavami A, Villanueva NL. Gluteal augmentation and contouring with autologous fat transfer: part I. Clin Plast Surg 2018;45(2):249–59.
7. Ghavami A, Villanueva NL, Amirlak B. Gluteal ligamentous anatomy and its implication in safe buttock augmentation. Plast Reconstr Surg 2018;142(2):363–71.
8. Frojo G, Halani SH, Pessa JE, et al. Deep subcutaneous gluteal fat compartments: anatomy and clinical implications deep subcutaneous gluteal fat compartments: anatomy and clinical implications. Aesthetic Surg J 2022;00(0):1–8.
9. Wall S. SAFE circumferential liposuction with abdominoplasty. Clin Plast Surg 2010;37(3):485–501.
10. Ramírez-Montañana A. Commentary on: deep subcutaneous gluteal fat compartments: anatomy and clinical implications. Aesthetic Surg J 2022;43(1):84–5.
11. Gonzalez R, Gonzalez R. Intramuscular gluteal augmentation: the XYZ method. Clin Plast Surg 2018;45(2):217–23.
12. Chávez FP, Gonzalez EAF, Guerrero ORR, et al. The perception of the ideal body contouring in Mexico. Plast Reconstr Surg - Glob Open 2020;1–6. https://doi.org/10.1097/GOX.0000000000003155.
13. Mendieta CG. Classification system for gluteal evaluation. Clin Plast Surg 2006;33(3):333–46.
14. Whipple LA, Fournier CT, Heiman AJ, et al. The anatomical basis of cellulite dimple formation: an ultrasound-based examination. Plast Reconstr Surg 2021;148(3):375e–81e.
15. Ramos-Gallardo G, Orozco-Rentería D, Medina-Zamora P, et al. Prevention of fat embolism in fat injection for gluteal augmentation, anatomic study in fresh cadavers. J Investig Surg 2018;31(4):292–7.
16. Abboud M, Geeroms M, El Hajj H, et al. Improving the female silhouette and gluteal projection: an anatomy-based, safe, and harmonious approach through liposuction, suspension loops, and moderate lipofilling. Aesthetic Surg J 2021;41(4):474–89.
17. Del Vecchio D, Wall S. Expansion vibration lipofilling: a new technique in large-volume fat transplantation. Plast Reconstr Surg 2018;141(5):639e–49e.

Combining Fat and Implants for Gluteal Augmentation

Alexander Aslani, MD, PhD

KEYWORDS

- Buttock augmentation • Buttock implants • Gluteal augmentation • Gluteal implant complications
- Gluteal implant revision • Gluteal implants

KEY POINTS

- Surgical anatomy for gluteal implant surgery.
- Dual-plane buttock implant pocket dissection, technical suggestion for safe and efficient hybrid gluteal augmentation surgery with both implants and fatgraftin.
- Possibilities of combine waist shaping liposculpture and expansion vibration lipofilling fat grafting.

 Video content accompanies this article at http://www.plasticsurgery.theclinics.com.

Gluteal augmentation is steadily increasing in patient demand as well as performed procedures. Large-volume fat grafting for reshaping and/or augmenting buttocks, the so-called BBL procedure, remains the most popular option.[1] According to data from the International Society of Aesthetic Plastic Surgery, on a global scale, 31,330 augmentation procedures involving implant placement have been performed.[2] Buttock implants are less frequently used, as many surgeons shy away from their use, and there is a common perception that buttock implants would be very prone to complications. It is impossible to deduce from the current statistics the number of hybrid buttock augmentation procedures performed, as gluteal augmentation procedures are reported as "fat grafting" or "implant-based," rather than "hybrid" in the society's survey. Combination procedures are not always differentiated. With growing popularity of hybrid buttock augmentation, statistics may one day specify and differentiate the various techniques surgeons used. The buttock implant procedure has been brandmarked with a disproportionally high complication rate, with published values exceeding 38%.[3] It seems reasonable to presume that this high complication rate may reflect surgeon inexperience with the buttock implant procedures, rather than inherent flaws of the operation.

Important advantages of using buttock implants include stable volume augmentation and creation of core projection. Furthermore, buttock implants are, in contrast to fat grafting only BBL, not associated with potentially lethal fat embolism. Fat embolism and the unfortunate downstream consequences have been a major safety concern in the plastic surgery community since its first description in 2015.[4] Safety precautions and techniques are active topics of discussion among experts of plastic surgery society task force groups and the media.

When combining gluteal implants and fat grafting, we generally prefer round implants, although use of anatomical implants has been described and is favored by others.[5] For optimum outcomes with best possible safety profile, we recommend the combination of cohesive silicone gel buttock implants together with large-volume "expansion vibration lipofilling" (EVL) fat grafting and have branded the hybrid approach "supercharged BBL." The original description of this technique was in 2019.[6] Hybrid buttock augmentation has

Cirumed Clinic Marbella, Edificio Panorama, Autovía del Mediterráneo, km 184, planta baja, local 2B y 2C, Marbella, Málaga 29603, Spain
E-mail address: aaslani@cirumed.es

Clin Plastic Surg 50 (2023) 563–571
https://doi.org/10.1016/j.cps.2023.05.001
0094-1298/23/© 2023 Elsevier Inc. All rights reserved.

also been described with syringe fat grafting technique.[7]

The most important key for success is achieving good soft tissue coverage over the implants. Thus, we suggest a dual-plane pocket technique, dissecting the cranial part of the pocket in a submuscular plane under gluteus maximus and gluteus medius muscles and transitioning to a deep intramuscular level when reaching the sciatic foramen. Dual-plane pocket dissection provides the thickest possible muscle coverage superiorly but also allows for a protective layer of muscle between the implant and sciatic nerve in the critical lower half of the pocket.[8]

The hybrid supercharged buttock augmentation technique is especially suitable for male to female gender reassignment[9] and is currently our first-line option for this patient collective. Description of submuscular approaches exist although we suggest that these in fact may refer to the concept of very deep intramuscular pocket dissection.[10,11] For an optimum outcome, we recommend supplemental fat transfer to the hips, along the lateral edge of the gluteal muscle. Also, if the patient presents with a significant lateral deficiency, it is critical to add volume to the trochanteric depressions. We endorse EVL, described by Del Vecchio and Wall,[12] as the most efficient and efficacious technique for this purpose.

SURGICAL TECHNIQUE
Step 1: Liposuction and Fat Grafting

We favor combination anesthesia with both general anesthesia in addition to a spinal block. We circumferentially scrub and prepare all surgical sites while patients are in the standing position in order place them directly on the operating room table/sterile field; this allows for the freedom to reposition patients intraoperatively without the need for additional supplies, which ultimately saves expenses and time. Surgery is started in the supine position for fat harvest and waist liposculpture. Liposuction technique depends on the preference of each surgeon. There is no evidence for superiority of any single technique over others. Our preference is vibration power–assisted liposuction with fat collection in single closed canister in a closed sterile circuit.

We typically start in the supine position with tumescent infiltration containing adrenaline and tranexamic acid but no lidocaine. Tumescent infiltration and fat equalization are performed with 5 mm or 4 mm basket cannula, shaping liposuction of the abdomen, and the flanks with 4 mm Mercedes cannula. Achieving a good result in gluteal augmentation translates to creating a feminine waist-to-hip ratio. Special emphasis is placed on shaping the area adjacent to the iliac crest, especially the fat pad below the crest, referred to as the BIC (below-iliac-crest) zone. Modest liposuction in this area contributes to the impression of a "shorter and rounder" buttock, whereas overzealous suctioning in this area can create a "subiliac-hollow" appearance; this is very difficult to correct and should be avoided. The exact amount of liposculpting is essential here (**Fig. 1**).

Fat grafting can be done before or after implant placement, alternatively both, so the larger amount of graft can be placed before implant placement. If sufficient fat is available, additional fat transfer can be performed to smooth transitions and make final shape adjustments after implants are in position.

Fig. 2 shows possible fat grafting areas in green and implant locations inside the gluteus muscle in purple color. The fat is injected into the marked areas by positioning the cannulas in the subcutaneous planes via small incisions made on the flanks and infragluteal folds. The preoperative topographic marking is key for the success of the fat transfer. During this process, graft is injected subcutaneously through several passes using the EVL technique. Care is taken to find the perfect balance between passes for vibration tissue expansion in order to loosen up the tissue scaffold accommodating fat infiltration without over dissection of the soft tissue support. We recommend focusing on the perigluteal areas lateral to the gluteus major muscle border and avoid the incisional zone for pocket access. Our aesthetic focus remains on grafting into the trochanteric depressions (hip dips) where volume replacement is highly desired, because traditional gluteal implants will not provide volume in this region. The liposuction/fat grafting technique is demonstrated in Video 1.

Step 2: Pocket Dissection and Implant Placement

A new sterile field is prepared before dissection is started. In addition, a betadine-soaked compress is sutured over the anus using a number 0 silk stitch, to achieve a watertight separation from the surgical field.

We perform ultrasound measurement of gluteus mayor muscle thickness and subcutaneous fat layer before pocket dissection. The procedure entails making a 5-cm skin incision on both sides of the intergluteal cleft. We favor a 2-incision access over a single gluteal cleft incision. The initial dissection is beveled, leaving adequate subcutaneous fat for closure and preserving the sacrocutaneous

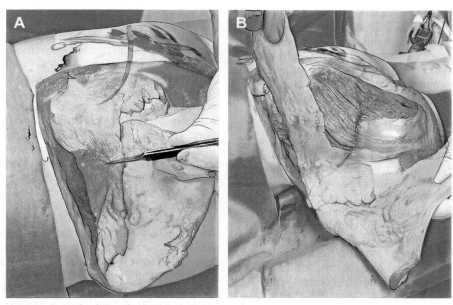

Fig. 1. (*A, B*) Dissection of subiliac fat pad in cadaver specimen.

ligament. The dissection proceeds until the gluteus maximus is identified, at which point direct access to the muscle fascia is created. In the cranial part of the incision, the muscle is split vertically, and a dissection clamp is pushed down to the concavity of the iliac bone shovel. Enough muscle dissection should be made to leave a thick muscle flap of around 3 cm. A blunt dissector is first used to create a submuscular space for the implant in the upper half of the implant pocket (Fig. 3). When the dissection approaches the height of the sciatic foramen, the dissector is beveled to a flatter angle to switch into an intramuscular plane (Video 2: Cadaveric dissection). Thus, the implant is submuscular in the cranial half of the pocket and intramuscular in

the lower half of the pocket, hence the term "dual-plane" (Video 3: Animation composite gluteal augmentation with dual-plane pocket).

To avoid the aesthetic complication of a high implant malposition, the surgeon needs to appropriately expand the tight ischiocutanous ligament in the lower pole of the pocket (Video 4: Sciatic release). A sterile surgical compress is immersed in adrenaline solution and placed inside the pocket during the dissection process to prevent excessive

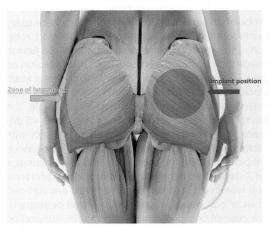

Fig. 2. Fat grafting areas in green and implant locations inside the gluteus muscle.

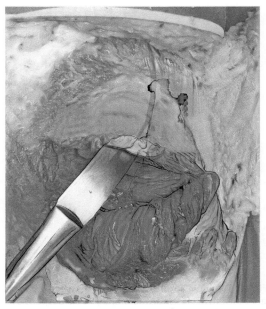

Fig. 3. Entry point into submuscular plane.

bleeding. In order to determine the ideal implant size, the surgeon can use an implant size as used for breast surgery. Alternatively, one can use soaked abdominal surgical compresses to determine pocket size. One abdominal compress corresponds to approximately 130 cc of volume. Determining accurate height and width of the implant ensures an adequate pocket is created to avoid the implant from rotating.

The implant insertion procedure begins with soaking the implant in an antibiotic solution. The implant is then inserted using the plastic funnel devices that have been sterilized. As a measure of preventing excessive fluid from accumulating in the pocket, a number 14 suction drain is placed in each pocket. It is important to double-check that the drain is not located directly on the central undersurface of the implant where it could possibly exert traction force to the sciatic nerve. Placing of final implants into the pockets is greatly simplified by using a sterile Keller funnel style plastic sleeve. For pocket closure, a dynamic suspension suture (Maxon size 0) is used to anchor each gluteal facia to its contralateral side to achieve mutual contralateral stabilization and avoid early gluteal implant ptosis (**Fig. 4**). The concept of mutual stabilization is similar to the columns of an "Arabic arch," and this is why it has been labeled "Arabic arch suture suspension." The subcutaneous layer is closed using a long-term absorbable monofilament suture, and a negative-pressure wound therapy device is used as a dressing for 7 days (**Figs. 5** and **6**).

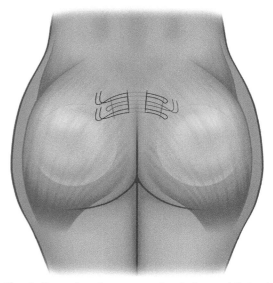

Fig. 4. Dynamic suture suspension between bilateral gluteal muscle fascia (Arabic arch, AASS suspension). AASS, Arabic arch suture suspension.

CHOICE OF IMPLANTS

In our practice, we exclusively use smooth cohesive silicone gel implants. As matters stand in 2023, these are not approved in the United States by the Food and Drug Administration (FDA). Hence, surgeons in the United States are limited to the use of solid elastomer silicone implants. Cohesive gel buttock implants come in 3 shapes: round, oval, or biconvex. We favor round implants for approximately 95% of our primary cases. Additional fat grafting gives the surgeon the possibility to alter the shape of soft tissues around the implants. Oval implants are attractive because they can give focused volume to the lower pole, but implant flipping is a problem that is challenging to manage without reoperation. Also, when using oval-shaped implants it is advisable to opt for textured-surface implants to reduce the risk of malrotation. Unfortunately, devices with a textured surface are more prone to seroma formation in the highly vascular gluteus muscle tissue. Biconvex implants provide very good projection but are only available in rather large sizes (above 370 cc) and can cause tissue thinning and atrophy. In slim-built patients with less muscle bulk they should be used with caution, as "soft tissue failure" is a risk factor.

The main objective when using buttock implants is to create projection, and round smooth will enable to achieve this sufficiently in most cases. Hip volume, or rather, filling out of trochanteric depressions, is created by EVL lipofilling. Soft tissue envelope thickening via fat grafting does also reduce visibility issues.

POSTOPERATIVE CARE

We routinely leave drains for a total of 7 days because fluid collections often peak after day 5. Ambulation is limited to the minimum necessary to prevent the implant displacement, seroma, rotation, and other complications. Especially hip flexion needs to be avoided because this brings tension on the dynamic suspension. Patients may use a foam block for "protected sitting." This means that when patients sit on a heightened surface (ie, the foam block) hip flexion is limited to less than 45 degrees. We recommend twice daily skin wash with Hibitane shower gel. Patients receive intravenous antibiotics during the procedure and oral antibiotics for 7 days after. Immediately after surgery and for 4 to 6 weeks afterward the patients are encouraged to wear compression garments. These postoperative restrictions prevent swelling while supporting the surgical areas to enhance patient comfort. Controlled, moderate-intensity stretching exercises

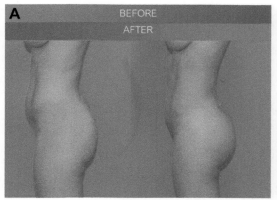
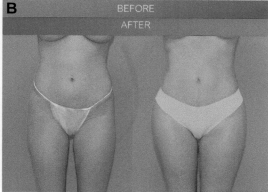
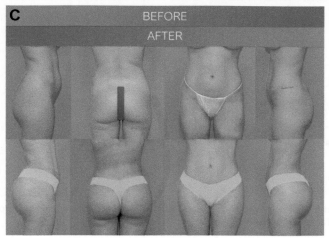

Fig. 5. (*A–C*) Before and after composite buttock augmentation 330 cc round smooth implants with dual-plane pocket, plus 400 cc EVL fat grafting on each side.

ease discomfort and speed up recovery. Regarding exercise after buttock implant surgery, we recommend to gradually increase intensity, at the earliest, 6 weeks after surgery and avoid abrupt overload. Stressing the gluteus muscle too early after surgery can lead to chronic inflammatory symptoms, which may prolong recovery and lead to irreversible damage.

Complications of Buttock Implants

The most frequent, although not necessarily the most relevant, complication in our patient collective are, usually minor, *wound healing problems* of the implant pocket incisions. We submit that one of the key advantages of using the double pocket incision is to maintain a layer of subcutaneous fat tissue padding under the incisions, facilitating secondary healing. Single midline incisions are more prone to proceed to grave problem because they do not have as much soft tissue padding.

Use of vacuum-assisted wound closure systems adapted for the use on skin incisions (3M

Prevena, España S.L.) for 7 days postop offers an additional, effective barrier to protect the incision during the initial wound healing phase. Including vacuum-assisted closure systems into our protocols has cut down our incidence of wound healing complications down to 8%, compared with 25% before its use.

The most relevant surgical complication of buttock implant surgery is *periprosthetic seroma* in the implant pocket. Seroma has been reported in literature as a frequent buttock implant complication.[13,14] We propose that the highly vascular thick muscle flap surrounding the implants may encourage seroma formation. A wound opening with serous drainage can be the first clinical sign and should always alert to screen for possible pocket seroma. We advise leaving suction drains for a minimum of 7 days. This period may seem long but helpful because patients are often significantly more mobile around day 5 postsurgery and are hence prone to develop a subacute seroma.

Infection in our experience is nearly always secondary due to an uncontrolled seroma. Drainage of

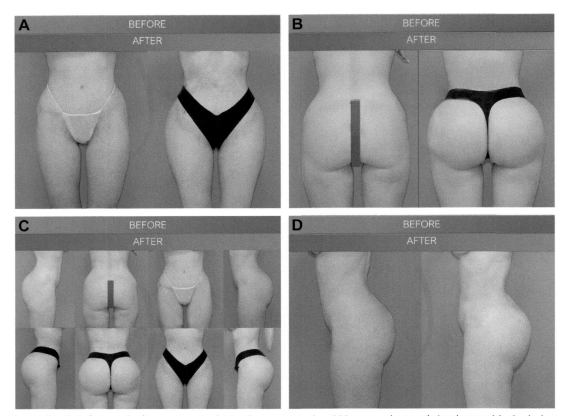

Fig. 6. (A–D) Before and after composite buttock augmentation 390cc round smooth implants with dual-plane pocket, plus 450cc EVL fat grafting each side.

seroma through a wound opening is an entry gate for possible infection. In our patient population, we observe a remarkably high resistance of buttock implants against infection. If infection is suspected in the presence of drainage, we recommend taking a bacteriology culture for targeted antibiotic treatment. If there are no progressive local infection signs (redness, fever) and infection parameters drop, conservative treatment is usually successful. Only if the patient develops fever with a sharp increase of infection parameters should the implants be removed.

Sciatic nerve damage is very rare and unlikely with correct and meticulous dissection technique. We recommend to always secure proper motoric function in recovery room by asking the patient to flex and extend the ankle as well as check sensitivity in the peroneal area; this documents there is no direct surgery-related traction injury to the nerve. Should any kind of sciatic neuropraxia symptoms occur in the recovery period, it is recommendable to rule out pressure of possible seroma via ultrasound. If a seroma cannot be identified, symptoms will in most cases be mild, attributable to swelling, and likely resolve with

resolution of swelling. Physiotherapy and stretching exercises are very helpful and recommended.

Capsular contracture is unusual and rare in buttock implant surgery. We are not aware of any cases that have been verified with histopathology. The lack of capsular contracture reports in the literature is a matter of debate; however, it seems reasonable to presume that the high vascularity of the gluteus muscles and the naturally high degree of mobility could explain this.

Animation deformity is not actually a complication, but rather, in most cases, a misperception. It is in the nature of an intramuscular implant pocket that implants will move to some degree with muscle contraction. It is also completely logical. Nevertheless, we do periodically see patients who are concerned with the upward displacement of implants on very forceful contraction, although this is actually a sign that implants are correctly positioned. We list this point here to stress the importance of patient education and setting appropriate expectations during the preoperative consultation.

Movement, malposition, and "flipping" of implants can be due to a variety of causes; both surgeon and/or patient factors can contribute to this complication. Iatrogenic causes include over-sizing of implants resulting in muscle atrophy and widening of the pocket or primary pocket overdis-section allowing for implant migration. Seromas can also be either a surgeon- or a patient-related issue. Surgeon error includes failure to use closed suction drains, whereas patient-related issues are due to postoperative instruction noncompliance—starting exercise and excessive movements too soon after surgery.

DISCUSSION OF CONTROVERSIES
Fat Grafting Before Versus After Implant Placement

We prefer to perform most of the fat grafting before redraping the patient and initiating the implant pocket dissection. A major advantage is that there are no concerns regarding accidental fat graft injection into the implant pocket. Getting optimal cannula angulation for precise fat grafting is easier and more efficient. Fat grafting with implants in place can inadvertently cause the surgeon to angle the cannula in potentially risky trajectories.

On the other hand, fat grafting after buttock implant placement may allow for more targeted and precise placement of the fat in areas that require the additional volume; this is a strong argument for after-buttock-implant placement, especially in patients with very deep trochanteric depressions or pronounced irregularities.

The wisest solution is to harness advantages from both approaches. The hybrid technique allows us to graft most of the fat before implant placement, and if sufficient fat is harvested, leave some for the fine-tuning adjustments after dissection of implant pockets and placement of the prothesis.

Choice of Dissection Plane

Currently accepted options for pocket dissection apart from our dual-plane technique are entirely intramuscular, entirely submuscular, and subfascial. The logic behind our recommended dual-plane technique is increased muscle tissue cover of the implants in the upper pole. The gluteus maximus muscle is not uniformly thick but has increasing thickness from cranial to caudal (Fig. 7). When dissecting a completely intramuscular pocket, the thin upper cranial third is a "weak point" prone to thinning of soft tissue envelope, implant edge visibility, and even herniation of implants. Recruiting additional gluteal medius fibers and staying completely submuscular enforce the pocket soft tissue cover in its weakest cranial part.

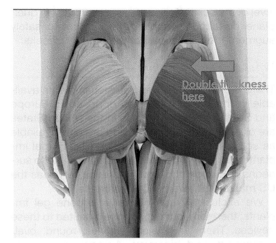

Fig. 7. Three different levels of gluteus mayor muscle thickness.

If one were to try creating a complete submuscular pocket, the dissection would be prematurely halted due to the inability to dissect caudal to the level of the sciatic foramen. The sciatic nerve exits through the foramen, and thus maintaining a submuscular plane below the upper edge of the sciatic foramen would endanger the nerve for traction or partial or complete transection injuries (**Fig. 8**). Given this limitation of dissection, purely submuscular implants result in a rather high implant position with flat lower buttock quadrants. Switching to the deep intramuscular below the

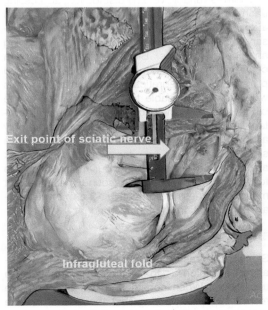

Fig. 8. Anatomical dissection of sciatic nerve through sciatic foramen.

level of the sciatic foramen, as we suggest in dual-plane dissection, enables the surgeon to safely augment the caudal part of the buttock cheeks.

What Are Different Implant Options?

There are key differences between implants available in the United States as opposed to Europe and South America. Implants in the United States are class II medical devices and are only available as solid block silicone. Cohesive silicone gel implants are class III devices and are available to surgeons in Europe and South America, whereas the US market still awaits FDA clearance.

We exclusively use cohesive silicone gel implants; therefore, our experience is limited to these devices. There are mainly 3 styles: round, oval/anatomical, and biconvex. Anatomical implants are designed for patients with long muscles and a high square buttock shape and round implants for patients with a rather short muscle.

When choosing the implant shape, it is important to remember that buttock implants are placed into a strong muscle with constant movement when patients are not just exercising but even when they are walking. Even with perfect implant placement, depending on patient physical activity, a moderate amount of muscle thinning can occur, allowing the implant to flip. With anatomical implants, the consequences can be catastrophic to say the least. Round-shaped implants are far more forgiving regarding this problem. When combining round implants with fat grafting, the surgeon has more freedom to variable volume distribution, addressing each patient's individual anatomy. Hybrid gluteal augmentation therefore makes it largely unnecessary to expose the patient to the problem of flipping anatomical implants. Biconvex implants have a convex shape on both sides, provide increased projection, and theoretically in case of flipping this would be unnoticeable to the patient due to the biconvex shape. They do, however, have an important limitation: currently biconvex implants are only available in sizes greater than 370 cc, which will be slightly oversized for most primary buttock augmentation cases. They are our implant of choice for very thick muscles (ultrasound measurement muscle thickness preoperative >3 cm) or secondary augmentation (implant exchange).

Benefit of Use of Drains

Similar to breast implant surgery, there is a variance of opinion as to whether it is beneficial to use drains. When considering this question, we recommend considering that the gluteal muscle is extremely vascular and even with limited patient mobility prone to seroma formation. Even minor seroma can create room for implant displacement and flipping. We therefore favor placement of size 14 redon drains. When placing drain tubes, make sure that drains are not placed directly underneath the implants where vacuum can possibly cause traction damage to the sciatic nerve. Regarding best time for removal, we have observed that patients tend to have significantly increased mobility from day 4 or day 5 onward. For our practice, we have determined day 7 after surgery as ideal time for drain removal.

SUMMARY

Composite (supercharged) gluteal augmentation is a very powerful tool in body contouring surgery. The 2 powerful techniques being combined are silicone implant placement and fat grafting, both when combined achieve strong core projection, waist shaping, and hip volume. We suggest dual-plane dissection and dynamic pocket suspension as 2 very strong assets to improve outcomes and reduce incidence of problems. The addition of fat transfer to the superficial subcutaneous layer avoids visibility of the implant contour in thin patients and, if enough fat graft as well as healthy recipient tissue availability, can achieve aesthetically very pleasing volume addition in the area of the trochanteric depression, leading to clearly better outcomes as compared with buttock implants alone.

CLINICS CARE POINTS

- Target points: key factor for success in buttock implant surgery is a pocket that is sufficiently deep to provide a robust and bulky soft tissue cover for buttock implants and at the same time leaves sufficient tissue between implant and muscle to protect the sciatic nerve. We present our strategy for progressive blunt instrument dissection as a time-efficient step-by-step approach to make buttock implants a reliable option for the body contouring surgeon's practice.
- We also share our technical suggestions for combination of hybrid surgery with large-volume fat grafting, which makes results more reliable by enhancing soft tissue cover and the outcome less dependent on the buttock implant only.

DISCLOSURE

The authors have nothing to disclose.

SUPPLEMENTARY DATA

Supplementary data related to this article can be found online at https://doi.org/10.1016/j.cps.2023.05.001.

REFERENCES

1. Sinno S, Chang JB, Brownstone ND, et al. Determining the safety and efficacy of gluteal augmentation: a systematic review of outcomes and complications. Plast Reconstr Surg 2016;137(4):1151–6.

2. Cárdenas-Camarena L, Trujillo-Méndez R, Díaz-Barriga JC. Tridimensional combined gluteoplasty: liposuction, buttock implants and fat transfer. Plast Reconstr Surg 2020;146(1):53–63.

3. Mofid MM, Gonzalez R, de la Peña JA, et al. Buttock augmentation with silicone implants: a multicenter survey review of 2226 patients. Plast Reconstr Surg 2013 Apr;131(4):897–901.

4. Deaths Caused by Gluteal Lipoinjection. What are we doing wrong? Plast Reconstr Surg 2015 Jul;136(1):58–66. Lázaro Cárdenas-Camarena 1, Jorge Enrique Bayter, Herley Aguirre-Serrano, Jesús Cuenca-Pardo.

5. Maltez G, Aboudib JH, Serra F. Long-term aesthetic and functional evaluation of intramuscular augmentation gluteoplasty with implants. Plast Reconstr Surg 2023;151(1):40e–6e.

6. Aslani A, Del Vecchio DA. Composite buttock augmentation: the next frontier in gluteal aesthetic surgery. Plast Reconstr Surg 2019;144(6):1312–21.

7. Miranda Godoy P. Alexandre mendonça munhoz 2 intramuscular gluteal augmentation with implants associated with immediate fat grafting. Clin Plast Surg 2018;45(2):203–15.

8. Aslani A, del Vecchio D, Bravo MG, Zholtikov V, Palhazi P. The dual-plane gluteal augmentation: an anatomical demonstration of a new pocket design. Plast Reconstr Surg 2023;151(1):45–50.

9. Del Vecchio D, Bravo MG, Mandlik V, et al. Body feminization combining large-volume fat grafting and gluteal implants. Plast Reconstr Surg 2022;149(5):1197–203.

10. Submuscular Gluteal Augmentation Jorge E. Hidalgo Clin Plast Surg 2018;45(2):197–202.

11. Petit F, Colli M, Badiali V. Buttocks volume augmentation with submuscular implants: 100 cases series. Plast Reconstr Surg 2022;149(3):615–22.

12. Vecchio DD, Wall S. Expansion vibration lipofilling: a new technique in large-volume fat transplantation. Plast Reconstr Surg 2018;141(5):639–49.

13. Senderoff D. Buttock augmentation with solid silicone implants. Aesthetic Surg J 2011;31(3):320–7.

14. Shah B. Complications in gluteal augmentation. Clin Plast Surg 2018;45(2):179–86.

Buttock and Full Body Contouring Harmony

Héctor César Durán Vega, MD[a,b,*]

KEYWORDS

- Buttock fat grafting • Brazilian butt lift • Liposuction • Liposculpture • Lipocontour • SIME • SIM3D

KEY POINTS

- Buttock surgery requires excellent anatomical knowledge.
- Buttock fat grafting is a safe procedure, with satisfactory results. However, the precise details must be considered to avoid complications.
- Fat infiltration should be performed in the subcutaneous space. Never intramuscular.
- Buttock volume is not enough. The shape is always as important as the volume and the buttock frame is as important as the buttock.
- Static injection migration and equalization or static injection migration and 3D superficial fat infiltration (SIM3D) should be considered as a safe and efficacious technique for fat buttock infiltration, providing projection and a round shape.

 Video content accompanies this article at http://www.plasticsurgery.theclinics.com.

INTRODUCTION

Buttock augmentation has been an increasing esthetic trend in most cultures, particularly in the West. Statistics reveal[1] an increase in the use of both fat and implants.

However, a phenomenon sometimes observed in esthetic surgery is that in the desire to improve on past results, one can sometimes push the boundaries too far. Such procedures produce results that cease to be esthetic or may even surpass the boundaries of what is considered normal. Therefore, the key to perform natural and beautiful buttock surgery lies in 4 elements: technology, anatomy, harmony (good relationship of the proportion of tissues), and surgical techniques to achieve it (Fig. 1).

A simple contribution is the concept of the gluteal frame. This allows surgeons to appreciate the relationship between the buttock and the rest of the body. This concept correctly applies the criteria of anatomy and harmony, allowing surgeons to choose the most appropriate technique. This has allowed us to know that a large buttock is not necessarily more beautiful but rather a buttock that relates appropriately proportionally to the surrounding frame.[2]

Finally, regarding surgical techniques, the most significant advancement of the last 5 years should be the progress in the safety of fat infiltration to the buttock. This has allowed us to modify the technique to minimize morbidity and avoid mortality.[3–9]

TECHNOLOGY IN BUTTOCK AUGMENTATION SURGERY

Ultrasonography

Ultrasound has become essential in many areas, especially in plastic surgery. It helps to prevent, diagnose, and treat various conditions and is especially useful in the buttock. The best ultrasound is the linear probe from 7 to 15 megahertz. This

[a] ASAPS, ASPS, AMCPER, FILACP, Centro Medico de Las Americas CMA, Consultorio#317 Calle 54 #365 x 33-a y Av. perez Ponce Colonia Centro, Merida, Yucatán CP 97000, Mexico; [b] Hospital Eme Red hospitalaria, Calle 33 Número 496, Consultorio 229, Entre 56 y 56 A, Centro, 97000 Mérida, Yucatán, México
* Hospital Eme Red hospitalaria, Calle 33 Número 496, Consultorio 229, Entre 56 y 56 A, Centro, 97000 Mérida, Yuc. México.
E-mail address: hcdv@hotmail.com

Clin Plastic Surg 50 (2023) 573–585
https://doi.org/10.1016/j.cps.2023.05.002

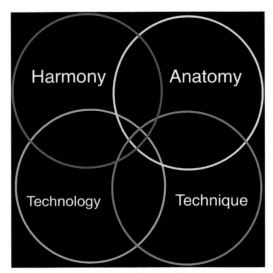

Fig. 1. The 4 core principles to achieve an adequate buttock contour.

type of configuration allows us to obtain more superficial images 4 to 9 cm deep, which is more than sufficient for fat infiltration. During fat infiltration surgery in the buttock, ultrasound helps to locate the deep subcutaneous space; thus, by placing the tip of the cannula, we can ensure that the infiltration is deposited in a location that will not cause problems[10] (Video 1).

Ultrasound Assisted Liposuction (UAL) (VASER or HEUS)

Both surgical devices use ultrasonic technology. The application of high-intensity ultrasound using sonotrodes generates emulsification of fat in the areas of liposuction and regularization; the difference being that VASER® (Solta Medical, Bothell, WA) is a third-generation device, and HEUS® (Indemex, Mexico and Dominican Republic) is the fourth-generation device, which produces the same effect but with a lower heat release. This allows the device to be used without ports because it does not heat or burn the skin, providing advantages in terms of speed and security. In addition, it has a special treatment called ultrasonic superficial optimizer (OSU), which allows the sonotrode to perform its function effectively without generating harmful temperature (Video 2).

The objective is to emulsify fat within the predetermined target area, translating to less surgeon fatigue in order to obtain fat by liposuction with less bleeding and a discreet effect of skin retraction. Its use is recommended, especially in high-definition areas, because it allows for a more straightforward definition and requires less effort

and decreased trauma to the body. It is especially useful when performing secondary liposuction as well as in tissues with increased fat density (such as in the male pectoral area). It is also considered that areas treated with ultrasound bleed less. There are 2 possible explanations for this finding. First, because the fat is emulsified, less trauma is required to extract the proper volume, which results in less trauma and therefore less bleeding. The second theory is that when performing the emulsification treatment, while passing the sonotrode a pretunneling is also being carried out, which allows a better distribution of the tumescence fluid, which improves the distribution of adrenaline within the tissues, allowing for increased vasoconstriction efficacy. However, using this technology augments the risk of seroma. Therefore, leaving a drain in treated areas is recommended.

Canister

Often times this topic is overlooked; however, the author thinks the specifics of where fat obtained will be deposited/stored are significant. The simplest method is to use a sterilized glass jar, wait for it to decant, strain the liquid obtained, and use the remaining fat yield. Multiple types of canisters exist; however, the characteristic that makes them worthwhile is proper isolation of fat. It is preferable that it has an adequate deposit volume with an egress valve in the dependent position to allow for efficient decanting of fluid. Various manufacturers produce canisters that meet these requirements.

Canisters that have a lower drain and allow the decanted liquid to exit through this hole also have the advantage of transporting fat to a pump for infiltration using the expansion vibration lipofilling (EVL) technique.[11,12] However, it is always necessary to check that the egress spout is of sufficiently large caliber (larger diameter than that of a Luer-Lock system) to prevent clogging of the harvested fat as it passes through the system.

Power assisted liposuction (PAL) (Microaire, Vibrasat, Others)

Performing liposuction with a vibrating device reduces the surgeon's push effort at the expense of device weight. This is the advantage of Microaire (MicroAire Surgical Instruments, Charlottesville, VA) compared with the others, which is much lighter and works very well, in addition to the diversity of cannula shapes and sizes. In addition to performing liposuction, the 4 or 5-mm basket cannulas can also be used for homogenizing irregular areas in a maneuver described as *SAFE*

Lipo by Wall.[13] The same set of cannulas and power-assisted device are also used with the EVL technique. This is an efficient method to infiltrate fat because a roller-pump controls the propulsion of fat through the entire system: Among the advantages of this technique are the speed of infiltration, the fact that the fat remains isolated from the environment, and it allows for adequate expansion of the treatment areas.[11]

Cannulas

When performing liposuction, the authors recommends the following modification to the Microaire cannulas. A proximal superior angulation, also named the "ergonomic Cannula" helps the surgeon move the cannula more efficiently and smoothly while decreasing the tension on the wrist and elbow. When surgeons use a straight cannula for liposuction, the tip can sometimes point in an unfavorable direction; therefore, they try to compensate for this by raising the tip. As a result, straight cannulas become curved after use. Using this modified cannula will be helpful, ergonomic, and practical because angulation allows for many versatile and safe movements[14] (Video 3).

Although multiple fat infiltration cannulas exist, the most helpful one is a 4 mm cannula with a single hole for the SIME technique (reviewed in more detail later). In this way, one can allow fat to flow appropriately without frequently becoming clogged (which often occurs when the cannula is 3 gauges or less). Some surgeons prefer 5-mm cannulas with more holes. However, new infiltration techniques allow for safer fat deposition in a single-depth plane, which benefits from the use of a single-hole cannula. Similarly, a basket cannula is helpful and generally used when performing EVL.

Infiltration cannulas with a Luer-Lock valve have several disadvantages. The risk of cannula misguidance has been previously described.[15] Moreover, the small diameter valve frequently becomes clogged, preventing constant laminar flow during fat infiltration. The base of the Toomey cannula had a larger diameter, facilitating better flow. However, its main drawback is that when attached to a syringe and lubricated with liquid and fat, it can loosen and dislodge. This is due to the positive pressure of the syringe, which can cause accidental spills and loss of valuable fat grafts. Therefore, an adequate cannula should be connected and securely locked allowing us to perform the proper movements without compromising safety (Video 4).

ANATOMY

Certain unsatisfactory results observed from patients presenting for revision and on social networks reveal that some surgeon do not respect or care for normal anatomy. Leaving esthetic canons can be rewarded by our patients in the short term, or even become a trend on social networks, but with time, they tend to lead to dissatisfaction. Eventually, patients will seek other surgeons to help them return to "normal." I strongly recommend maintaining our patients with a normal range in terms of volume and shape, with anatomic boundaries being our guiding light.

The gluteus can be analyzed using 2 anatomical criteria. The descriptive anatomy considers each single element, and the surface anatomy considers the entire area, considering the buttock rather than the gluteus maximus muscle (**Fig. 2**). Both are equally useful in designing our surgical plan.

When infiltrating fat into the buttock, the surgeon must consider a critical element, the subcutaneous cellular tissue, which should not be seen as a single structure but rather composed of 2 elements that can be used differently. It should be noted that these are 2 very distinct anatomic areas, the superficial and deep subcutaneous cellular tissues, divided by the fascia superficialis, which isolates and limits both locations along the entire length of the buttock, particularly in young patients. This effective isolation and integrity may sometimes be lost in older patients or in patients with enormous weight loss owing to a lack of tissue turgor.[16]

The superficial subcutaneous space is immediately underneath the skin (**Fig. 3**). This space comprises multiple septa in a swarm of connective tissues that allow the skin to be adequately fixed. If we advance a cannula through this area, we see that the skin retracts and wrinkles as it passes, which allows us to indirectly confirm its location and depth at that moment (Video 5). It has small spaces in which fat is very compact and does not accommodate much volume. If we attempt to infiltrate this area with high pressure and volume, lumps of fat are usually observed through the skin. If we abuse its capacity, the result will be a square plate by the infusion of excess fat, which is flat and too complex to mold to obtain a curved appearance.

Conversely, the deep subcutaneous space, bound by the superficial fascia superficially and the gluteus maximus fascia deep, has a much more potential capacity for expansion that allows for a greater volume of infiltrated fat. I have found that this is the better area to inject fat because it will make the buttocks rounder and more projected while controlling fat volume. The main advantage is that the fat that enters this area is safe without the risk of muscle infiltration (Video 5).

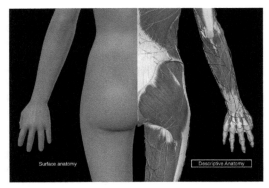

Fig. 2. Differences between surface anatomy, which observes the buttock as a unit, and descriptive anatomy that observes each part of the whole in segments.

Fat can successfully infiltrate the subcutaneous space, increasing the volume of the buttock, as previously demonstrated.[6,9] The gluteus maximus muscle is located deep to the targeted zone. It is vital to avoid infiltration with fat, even superficially, because its migration capacity can direct fat to the deep subgluteal space, thereby enhancing its volume and pressure. This can theoretically pull and injure the gluteal venous vessels by traction in the emerging foramen, causing macroscopic fat embolism (MAFE).[3–5,7,8,17] Therefore, the muscle should not be infiltrated. Caution regarding the danger of injury to the gluteal blood vessels located in the submuscular space, based on the anatomical area in which they are located (described as the "danger triangle")[18] becomes unnecessary when we understand that infiltration must occur in the subcutaneous cellular tissue. Thus, the infiltrated area is irrelevant if it is superficial and not muscular. The fat should never be

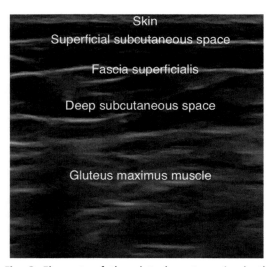

Fig. 3. Elements of the gluteal anatomy in depth observed by means of a linear ultrasound.

injected at a depth that involves the gluteus maximus.

Considering the necessity for a high degree of safety, we must provide plastic surgeons who have a limited experience in these procedures with a reference on how to achieve esthetically pleasing and harmonious results while restricting fat transfer to the subcutaneous space. Harnessing various benefits of the distinct subcutaneous spaces one can optimize shape while augmenting volume.

HARMONY

All plastic surgeons should appreciate the concept of harmony to deliver both normal and natural volumes. Therefore, plastic surgeons possess the responsibility to avoid creating a new species of human anatomy. Simply giving volume to the buttock is insufficient; each zone must be precisely addressed creating contrast between areas of concavity and convexity in a way that is esthetically pleasing. Anatomy guides surgeons because it is the only constant between patients of various shapes and sizes. In summary, harmony in body contours consists of achieving a good relationship between the volume and shape of the anatomical areas, so that the result is esthetic and natural. It can only be created correctly if the anatomy is respected and maintained.

The buttocks are round mounds, a three-dimensional area of convexity between the lower back and upper thighs. However, we must remember that the goal is to recreate the shape achieved by the gluteus maximus muscle. Therefore, the entire buttock cannot be augmented evenly. The rectangular muscle originates in the sacrum and inserts onto the trochanter and iliotibial tract. To achieve a proper anatomical shape, the inner lower region usually does not infiltrate.

The relationship between the waist and hip is usually described as a ratio of 0.7 to 0.6, as well as the buttock and leg (according to Singh's article[19,20] on the relationship of tissue proportions). The psychologist Singh affirms that this is the "ideal" proportion, which is considered attractive to human beings regardless of culture. We invite readers to read the studies of different relationships between the anatomical areas.[21–24] However, very often, the result between the dimensions of the tissues range from 0.7 to 0.65 (buttock-leg, waist, hip, and so forth) depending on patient desires or the surgeons artistic eye.

Laterally, the area we want to augment the most corresponds to point c of Mendieta landmark article,[2] which lies at approximately the level of the greater trochanter. Marking it preoperatively allowed us to accurately locate it regardless of intraoperative patient positioning. However, fat is carefully grafted such that the newly created point of maximal projection maintains a continuous, gentle transition to the thigh. A small, lateral concavity corresponds to vertical and inferior displacement of the iliotibial tract between the gluteal muscle and the hip. This trait is appreciated in athletic and thin patients but not necessarily in those to whom we want to give more volume or have a mass index greater than 25. No grooves were observed in these cases.

Achieving a rounded, esthetically pleasing gluteal augmentation result requires working well on the entire aspect of the frame. Mendieta showed us that the lateral frame is optimized by looking for the A or curved aspect[2]; however, until now, the gluteal frame has only been considered in terms of how the hip influences the shape. However, the current framework is composed of the sacrum, supragluteal region, spine, hip, infragluteal groove, and superior thigh.[25,26] The paravertebral muscles should be delimited with the midline marked in the sacrum area and a small channel that extends from the intergluteal site to both sides in the form of butterfly wings, which have the dimples of Venus as the upper limit.

All areas surrounding the buttock and its structures (ie, muscles and fascia, fat, and skin) are prone to change. Each structure can exhibit deficiencies, alterations, or inadequate harmony/balance.

AVOIDING BUTTOCK-THIGH DISPARITY

One of the most frequently observed problems in buttock surgery is when the surgeon considers the buttock to be an isolated structure. In normal anatomy, a bulky or muscular buttock is always accompanied by an equally strong or bulky thigh (hamstrings posteriorly and quadriceps femoris anteriorly). One should always consider placing fat in the transition between the buttock and thigh to avoid this disparity, and the key site is an infragluteal fold. Thus, an elongated fold beyond the midline should always be avoided. It must be ensured that it has adequate angulation with a beautiful transition lateral to the midgluteal spot. In a previous publication, we refer to this as "vectorial treatment of the infragluteal fold," a way to work correctly address deformities in that area.[27] The posterior portion of the thigh is augmented in parallel for balance.[28]

THE TECHNIQUE

For this technique, I recommend reviewing what has been written about Lipocontour.[25,26,29] This

form of standardized preoperative marking guides us by utilizing the underlying anatomy as a roadmap. Although the patient is placed in different positions throughout the operation, we can continue the liposuction, knowing which areas have been addressed and avoid overzealous suction and dermal injury. This also helped standardize results.

Once fat is harvested with liposuction, it is decanted in the closed canister. If the canister has an inferiorly places egress valve, all seroussanguinous fluid is drained. If the canister lacks a valve in the dependent position, we remove the decanted fluid by aspiration from a thin (3 mm) liposuction cannula. Once fat reaches the cannula, it becomes clogged, indicating that the fluid had been adequately evacuated. Once all of the fat is isolated, it is placed in 60-mL syringes (Video 4). We then proceeded with infiltration.

Infiltration incisions: Generally, incisions are made in the upper part of the intergluteal groove, infragluteal folds, hip, and sometimes at the peak of each buttock. The last incision is disadvantageous from an esthetic perspective because it can be easily seen. Nevertheless, this is beneficial when working on the waist and infiltrating the buttocks.

Liposculpture is performed in 4 positions: front, back, and sides. During the last year and a half, I have changed my practice and now infiltrate the gluteus from the lateral position; it has provided outstanding results because it allows observation of tissue responsiveness as fat is grafted and how it responds in real-time to the infiltration (Videos 4 and 6). However, I finalize and execute final refinements with the patient in the prone position. I have found that this enables me to improve projection in a more balanced manner. In general, the practice limits fat liposuction to no more than 5 L. The infiltrated volume on average per buttock, and the hip ranges from 750 to 1000 cc per side. Almost half of this volume goes into the infiltration of the hips and legs and the other half into the buttock.

CONSTRUCTION OF BUTTOCKS WITH FAT INFILTRATION

There is not universally accepted or foolproof method to infiltrate fat into the buttocks and achieve good results. The pleasant appearance of the buttock depends not only on its volume but also on the shape of the buttock and the surrounding area. However, achieving excellent buttock results usually requires the grafting of large volumes. The main challenge when infiltrating fat is to achieve a round buttock with proper projection and shape. When surgeons inject fat indiscriminately with the goal of increasing volume, we have observed that this does not necessarily correct shape. This becomes problematic especially in patients who desire a rounder shape but present with an already fat-filled square buttock because it accepts less fat infiltration in areas that need it most. The first thing that is built is the volume and projection, and the last is the shape, which sometimes may require additional liposuction or internal ligamentous releases.

STATIC INJECTION MIGRATION AND EQUALIZATION AND SIM3D

Dr Dan del Vecchio is credited for publishing the Static Injection Migration and Equalization (SIME) technique; a handy and safe tool incorporated into the fat infiltration portion of buttock augmentation procedures.[30] SIME are the steps to safely and efficiently infiltrate fat into the buttocks. To summarize, the deep subcutaneous space must be identified using ultrasonography during surgery, and the tip of the infiltration cannula should be correctly positioned in the deep fat compartment. It remains static during fat infiltration. It is important to locate the best place for SIME. We do this by identifying the area with the most significant gluteal volume deficit and starting infiltrating a volume of 120 to 180 cc (Video 7).

Once infiltrated, we can appreciate how the fat is distributed based on internal pressure/resistance gradients creating passive diffusion. The surgeon can reinject fat into the same deep space but in a different place. The advantage of identifying the space using ultrasound is that the surgeon can perform infiltration during cannula recoil, knowing that it will not violate the facia and inadvertently infiltrate fat into a dangerous area. Once infiltration is completed in 2 or 3 SIME sites, equalization can be performed with a 4-mm basket cannula to disperse the fat more homogeneously. This maneuver changes the internal subcutaneous structure creating additional capacitance for fat to migrate to and fill in. Ultimately, this allows the surgeon to affect external buttock contours by manipulating internal fat positioning. With ultrasound, we can corroborate that the fat migrates in the subcutaneous space laterally but respects the deep facial plane preventing fat migration into the muscle. It also generally respects the superficial space if it has not been previously damaged/violated. Some publications warn against this method of bolus infiltration[8,31] due to a high risk of complications, including a lack of fat integration, oily cysts, seromas, and even abscesses; evidence has shown that this is not the case. Ultrasonographic studies were performed on more than 35 patients who underwent this technique with a follow-up period of up to 6 months. None of the patients had significant infection, seroma, or cyst. (The only cyst I have been able to document was a small 2-mm cyst.) A few cases are still being studied; however, thus far, the results have been satisfactory and without problems. I think this is mainly due to the ability of fat to migrate at the level of deep subcutaneous cellular tissue,[9] which allows the infiltrated fat to spread and does not remain a single isolated bolus of fat. Proper equalization techniques and manual massage allows for dispersion of fat between tissues to increase integration capacity.

Figs. 4–7 show before and after buttock fat infiltration with SIM3D.

Fat infiltrates all surrounding tissues in the deep subcutaneous infiltration and compartments.[32] To obtain adequate projection and shape, the surgeon might perform anywhere from 2 to 4 different SIME deposits according to the buttock projection needs. It is important to always use ultrasound-guided visualization of the cannula to confirm the depth of fat grafting. The last SIME step involves of equalization (Video 6), which is the dispersion of the infiltrated fat with a 4 or 5 mm basket cannula so that the fat is better distributed. I have found that this last step is not always necessary and should be used cautiously because it helps in the distribution of fat but also reduces the projection achieved with this technique. That is why I recently began performing SIM3D. After performing SIM (without the E for equalization), the three-dimensional (3D) technique is performed, which is a technique of infiltration of the subcutaneous superficial space in small volumes like using a 3D printer (hence the name) to shape better the buttock. When a 3D printer works, it make a long journey with the printer head (in this case, the infiltration cannula) but the material is only deposited in small parts in the areas objective, according to the shape you want to give it. Similarly, when infiltrating fat, although the cannula moves in large routes, we only infiltrate the fat in the areas in which we want to provide more volume selectively and, thus, achieve a more esthetic and rounder buttock (Video 8).

The relative amount of fat infiltrated during each portion of the procedure approximates 75% SIM and 25% 3D. It is important to highlight 2 essential characteristics of this technique: fat deposition is always carried out within the superficial subcutaneous tissue and fat deposition is carried out in small quantities at low pressure. We recommend that fat deposition be performed by squeezing the syringe gently, accompanying the movement of the cannula, with the fat flowing naturally,

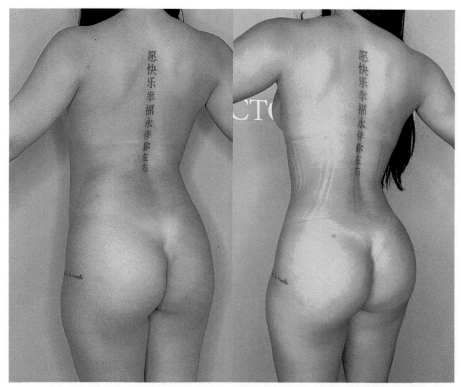

Fig. 4. A 23-year-old woman, 6 months after surgery. We observed more defined and narrower waist according to Lipocontour marking, decrease in sacral volume, and increase in gluteal volume with the SIM3D technique.

accompanying the movement without exerting excessive pressure. In this manner, we can achieve a good area shape and create a round contour. As mentioned previously, a 4 to 5-mm single-hole cannula is recommended for SIM so that we know exactly where we are placing the fat; for 3D, we recommend that a 3 to 4-mm cannula of 3 or 4 cross holes be used so that the dispersion is greater.

Although the size of the subcutaneous space can vary from patient to patient due to age, sex, and other variables,[16] the fascia superficialis consistently separates the deep and superficial subcutaneous spaces. When the tumescent solution infiltrates into the deep space, the superficial fascia effectively isolates the spaces, preventing fluid flow into the surface space. SIM3D fat transfer allows fat to be placed in an optimized manner, understanding the histological characteristics of each site and, at the same time, making it safe.

Generally, 50% of the infiltration volume of the buttock is performed in the prone position, and the other 50% in the lateral decubitus position (25% per side). The lateral position allows for one to appreciate volume deficiencies in different areas, which usually requires more volume in the lower and lateral gluteal areas. I usually place more fat in this area and the hip.

Once the necessary fat is grafted, a closed suction drain is placed in the subcutaneous space existing from the sacrum and a second one in the abdominal area for 7 days. All incisions are closed with a single or X-spot of vicryl rapid 3-0, so there is no need to be removed. Bandages and cotton are placed for comfortable compression in the abdominal area, whereas there is no compression placed on the buttock area. The patient goes to the recovery area, where she will recuperate from anesthesia, and once fully improved, with tolerance of fluids, they can go home. The postoperative instructions for the patient include a regular diet, antibiotics, and analgesics for one week.

Figs. 8 and **9** show immediate postoperative result.

POSTOPERATIVE CARE

When performing any flap (tissue transfer procedure) in reconstructive plastic surgery, we avoid tight high-compression bandage. Therefore, why should high compression be indicated in

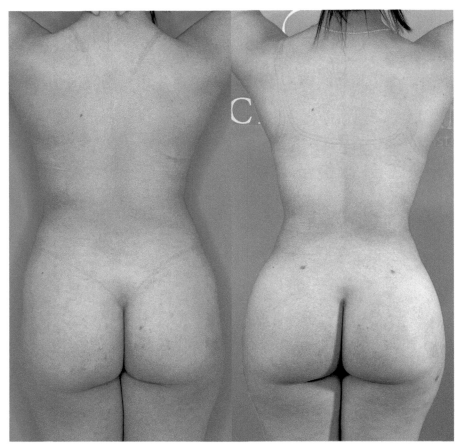

Fig. 5. A 22-year-old woman was 6 months after SIM3D and Liipocontour surgery. It is observed more narrower waist, decrease of fat of the back, the volume is increased with fat in the point c of Mendieta, and the gluteal volume is increased.

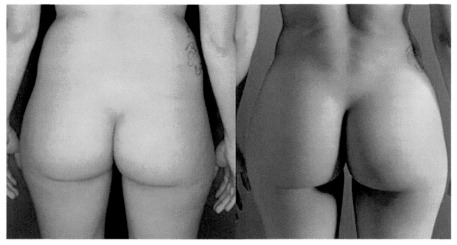

Fig. 6. A 34-year-old woman to 1 year of SIME and Lipocontour surgeries. It is observed better definition of the waist, anatomical marking of the area of the sacrum, increased gluteus and fat was placed in the waist, and the vector technique was used to improve the infragluteal groove.

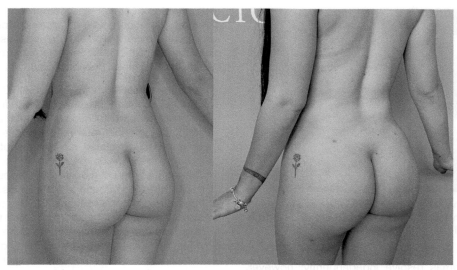

Fig. 7. A 27-year-old woman to 6 months of surgery. We observed better definition of the waist with Lipocontour, placement of fat in leg, and increase of buttock technique SIME.

liposuction flaps? Therefore, I usually put cotton and bandages on patients for a week, and subsequently recommend compression garments. I also asked patients not to lean or sit on the buttock area for 2 to 3 weeks, which, in theory will maintain a better shape of the buttocks. Unless contraindicated due to concomitant surgery of the anterior torso, they are asked to rest, sleep, and lay down in the prone position at home. If they undergo a tummy tuck or breast augmentation, they are advised to lie on their back but with a pillow that serves as a support on the lower back and leg, which relieves weight and direct pressure on the buttock. The patients are only allowed to sit when using the bathroom. A handy tool is a cushion that helps patients sit on the thigh, releasing pressure to the buttocks, which they are instructed to use for 3 weeks.

After 3 weeks, the patients are allowed to sit on their buttocks. For many years, I allowed the patients to sit on their buttocks immediately and lie on their backs without any restrictions, even immediately after the surgery. Although I did not observe major complications, I did notice a flattened appearance and loss of projection at the 3-week follow-up visit. Thus, I initiated these restrictions. The main esthetic advantage I observe is the maintenance of the projection and the rounded shape of the gluteal projection.

It also indicated antibiotics (usually levofloxacin) for a week after surgery and analgesic medications. After this week, diosmin-hesperidin may have improved inflammation.

Generally, a closed-suction drain is placed in the subcutaneous space for areas of liposuction—an anterior drain exits through one of the inguinal post sites and the posterior drain is placed through the sacral port site. This closed drainage system has the advantage of allowing the quantification of drainage, observation of the characteristics and volume of the drained drainage, and avoidance of contamination. In general, we removed it within 1 week of surgery.

COMPLICATIONS

Although it is generally considered safe, potential complications have resulted from the procedure, as with any surgical procedure. A complication of fat infiltration in the buttocks is the development of fat necrosis. The formation of nodules under the skin is caused by fat cell death and calcification. This can cause pain and discomfort, resulting in an uneven or lumpy appearance of buttocks. Although this complication is not life threatening, it can be esthetically displeasing, and in severe cases, surgical removal of necrotic tissue may be necessary.

Another possible complication of fat infiltration into the buttocks is infection.[33] The infection of the incision site can occur either naturally or accidentally when bacteria is introduced into the subcutaneous space during the procedure. Infections can be treated using antibiotics. In severe cases, it may be necessary to perform surgical intervention to drain the infected area.

Seroma formation is another potential complication after fat infiltration into buttocks. Swelling and discomfort can be caused by a seroma, which is a collection of fluids that can occur after surgery.

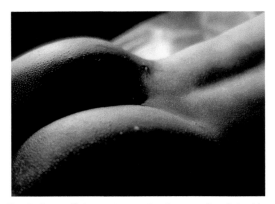

Fig. 8. Immediate postoperative image of a gluteal increase with fat infiltration with SIM3D and Lipocontour technique.

Most seromas resolve independently; however, ultrasound-guided puncture or surgical drainage may be necessary in severe cases.

When fat is treated with care and sterility during the procedure is not compromised, complications are infrequent, despite the large volume of fat that is being transferred. It is crucial to carefully follow all postoperative instructions to minimize the risk of complications. Patients should also immediately report any symptoms or concerns to their surgeons to ensure prompt and appropriate treatment.

Aesthetic Complications

So far, the only uncertainty in fat infiltration and what can be considered a consequence rather than a complication is the loss of volume during 6 months after fat infiltration. The volume is reabsorbed, and although no study has defined the extent to which it is absorbed, it is generally considered that approximately 40% to 50% of the infiltrated fat is lost.

Other esthetic complications of importance include a lack of adequate projection of the

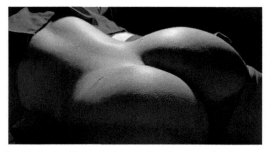

Fig. 9. Immediate postoperative image of a buttock augmentation with fat infiltration with SIM3D and Lipocontour technique.

gluteus anteroposterior and complications in the 4 corners. The 4 corners that fail are buttock areas with specific related problems, which is usually the main reason patients are present to my office dissatisfied with their previous results (**Fig. 10**).

1. Superio-medial corner (Region A): Generally, this area is not adequately filled with fat, which does not generate fullness or contour. It usually occurs if the upper intergluteal area is used as an approach because fat comes out quickly through the incision owing to its contiguity. This can easily be resolved by properly infiltrating the area through a distant incision.

2. Inferio-medial corner (Region B). This area represents a congenital anatomic variant that corresponds to a bulge that some patients present with (colloquially referred to as "dirty diapers"). Excess tissue makes the buttocks seem square and irregular, exacerbated by a strong ischial cutaneous ligament.[34] This can be solved by using a 4 to 5-mm basket cannula to release the ligament attached to the skin, applying energy, usually a laser or VASER, or taking the excess volume. It is common to not completely solve this if the problem is big. Therefore, direct skin resection should be considered.

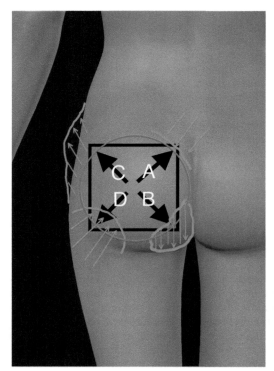

Fig. 10. The 4 corners deficits. Elements that are improperly treated after an infiltration of fat into the buttock.

3. Superio-lateral corner (Region C): This area most frequently generates problems because there is usually a lack of liposuction in the tissue above or below the edge of the iliac crest. Therefore, the gluteal frame was inadequate. This problem can be avoided through the guidance of the Lipocontour line (Video 9). The line in the anterior abdomen corresponds to the inguinal fold. Behind the highest point of the intergluteal line, 2 transverse lines were drawn, which, when joined laterally, always corresponded to the inguinal lines, forming a slight angulation. This line is essential because it properly demarcates the boundary between the waist and hip. Above this line, the volume should always be aspirated and decreased, and below, the volume should always increase until reaching the lateral zenith corresponding to point C of the Mendieta or trochanter, where there should be more significant lateral expansion. With this guide, it is very difficult to lose sight of the target, and it will always help the surgeon to guide the patient in a lateral position. Anatomically, it corresponds to approximately 2 to 4 cm below the edge of the iliac crest at the height of a vertical line drawn from the axillary line posterior to the middle of the thigh.

4. Inferio-lateral corner (region D), usually corresponds to a depression in the buttock that is not sufficiently filled by fat infiltration and leaves a V-buttock appearance. Vector treatment of this area will help avoid this, especially in the vertical and oblique approaches. However, it is common to find difficulties with its expansion. The solution is to infiltrate the appropriate fat volume, which is often more significant than initially considered by the surgeon.

Careful consideration of these boundaries coupled with calculated intraoperative maneuvers described above prevents postoperative deformities and optimizes results when molding buttocks.

PATIENT SELECTION AND THE PREOPERATIVE EVALUATION/CONSULTATION

Who should decide between buttock and full-body contouring? Is this only when a patient requests a total body transformation or is it the surgeon's preference to suggest additional contouring areas?

This is a delicate balance among the patient's desire, artistic appreciation of the surgeon, and patient's health and financial burden. On many occasions, the surgeon will know what to do to

achieve harmony in the patient's body but will need the right conditions to achieve it (eg, hemoglobin levels, fat available with low body mass index [BMI]).

It is necessary to guide the patient to what might deliver a more anatomical and beautiful result, which will always depend on the underlying anatomy of the patient. Sometimes, a small change or addition can achieve a spectacular result. On other occasions, this is impossible because the required surgery exceeds the safety level that can be provided to the patient. Therefore, it is not only a decision based on the patient's or the surgeon's desire but also on what can be done according to the patient's anatomy and physiologic condition. However, if possible, I think that the proper balance lies in listening to the patient's general desire, explaining what is best to achieve his dream according to our diagnosis and artistic ability, and in the end, in the decision of an informed patient, because it is their body, and we must respect the decision. If we disagree with the patient's decision, we should respectfully inform the patient and refer to another qualified surgeon.

SUMMARY

In conclusion, buttock augmentation has become a popular trend in many cultures, particularly in the West, with increasing use of both fat and implants. However, similar to any esthetic surgical procedure, it is essential to avoid exaggerated contours by excessive procedures, fat evacuation and fat grafting, which can result in unappealing or grossly abnormal appearing outcomes. To achieve a beautiful buttock, it is essential to consider the elements of technology, anatomy, harmony, and the appropriate surgical techniques. The concept of the gluteal frame has been a valuable addition to understanding the relationship between the buttock and rest of the body, allowing surgeons to choose the most appropriate technique for each patient. In addition, the safety of fat infiltration into the buttocks has significantly improved recently, allowing for modifications to the technique and avoiding potential problems. The construction of a round-projected buttock with fat infiltration is challenging. Although the volume of fat injected plays a crucial role in achieving a substantial buttock result, the shape of the surrounding area is crucial for a pleasant appearance. In our experience, building the volume and projection of the buttock is performed first, followed by the shape. Using ultrasound to identify the deep subcutaneous space, the SIME technique helps achieve safe and good gluteal volume and projection. The 3D technique helps obtain a better buttock shape by depositing a small volume in areas requiring complementary infiltration. In summary, buttock augmentation can produce esthetically pleasing results when appropriate elements are considered and applied correctly.

CLINICS CARE POINTS

- Use technology. It will make your surgery easier and safer, especially the use of imaging ultrasound.
- For a beautiful and natural buttock augmentation outcome, relay in the anatomy, both superficial and descriptive. The anatomy should always influence us because this is constant from patient to patient and serves as a guide.
- Always avoid fat infiltration in the muscle.
- SIME is the safest fat infiltration technique available now.
- SIM3D is a complementary technique for shape a round buttock. It is still safe because it is based on superficial fat infiltration along with the deep SIME fat infiltration. SIME gives projection and volume and 3D provides the shape.

DISCLOSURE

The author declares has nothing to disclose.

SUPPLEMENTARY DATA

Supplementary data related to this article can be found online at https://doi.org/10.1016/j.cps.2023.05.002.

REFERENCES

1. Available at: https://www.isaps.org/media/vdpdanke/isaps-global-survey_2021.pdf. Accessed March 5, 2023.
2. Mendieta CG. Classification system for gluteal evaluation. Clin Plast Surg 2006;33(3):333–46.
3. Bayter-Marin JE, Cárdenas-Camarena L, Aguirre-Serrano H, et al. Understanding fatal fat embolism in gluteal lipoinjection: a review of the medical records and autopsy reports of 16 patients. Plast Reconstr Surg 2018;142(Issue 5):1198–208. Lippincott Williams and Wilkins.
4. Cárdenas-Camarena L, Bayter JE, Aguirre-Serrano H, et al. Deaths caused by gluteal lipoinjection: what are we doing wrong? Plast Reconstr Surg 2015;136(1):58–66.
5. Cárdenas-Camarena L, Durán H, Robles-Cervantes JA, et al. Critical differences between microscopic (MIFe) and macroscopic (MAFE) fat embolism during liposuction and gluteal lipoinjection. Plast Reconstr Surg 2018;141(4):880–90.
6. del Vecchio DA, Villanueva NL, Mohan R, et al. Clinical implications of gluteal fat graft migration: a dynamic anatomical study. Plast Reconstr Surg 2018;142(5):1180–92.
7. Durán H, Cárdenas-Camarena L, Bayter-Marin JE, et al. Microscopic and macroscopic fat embolism: solving the puzzle with case reports. Plast Reconstr Surg 2018;142(4):569E–77E.
8. Ramos-Gallardo G, Durán-Vega HC, Cárdenas-Camarena L. Complications of gluteal fat augmentation. In: Cansanção A, Condé-Green A, editors. Gluteal fat augmentation: best practices in brazilian butt lift. Swizerland: Springer International Publishing; 2021. p. 151–5. https://doi.org/10.1007/978-3-030-58945-5_22.
9. Wall S, Delvecchio D, Teitelbaum S, et al. Subcutaneous migration: a dynamic anatomical study of gluteal fat grafting. Plast Reconstr Surg 2019;143(5):1343–51.
10. Mortada H, Al Mazrou F, Alghareeb A, et al. Overview of the role of ultrasound imaging applications in plastic and reconstructive surgery: is ultrasound imaging the stethoscope of a plastic surgeon? A narrative review of the literature. Eur J Plast Surg 2023;46:15–24.
11. del Vecchio D, Wall S. Expansion vibration lipofilling: a new technique in large-volume fat transplantation. Plast Reconstr Surg 2018;141(5):639e–49e.
12. del Vecchio D, Wall S, Stein MJ, et al. Simultaneous separation and tumescence: a new paradigm for liposuction donor site preparation. Aesthetic Surg J 2022;42(12):1427–32.
13. Wall SH, Lee MR. Separation, aspiration, and fat equalization: SAFE liposuction concepts for comprehensive body contouring. Plast Reconstr Surg 2016;138(6):1192–201.
14. Durán H, Pazmiño P. The proximal superiorly angled liposuction cannula. Plast Reconstr Surg 2021;148(1):161e–2e.
15. del Vecchio D, Kenkel JM. Practice advisory on gluteal fat grafting. Aesthetic Surg J 2022;42(9):1019–29.
16. Frank K, Casabona G, Gotkin RH, et al. Influence of age, sex, and body mass index on the thickness of the gluteal subcutaneous fat: implications for safe buttock augmentation procedures. Plast Reconstr Surg 2019;144(1):83–92.
17. Cárdenas-Camarena L, Durán-Vega HC, Ramos-Gallardo G, et al. Mortality following gluteal fat augmentation: physiopathology of fat embolism. In:

Cansanção A, Condé-Green A, editors. *Gluteal fat augmentation*. Cham, Switzerland: Springer; 2021. p. 145–9. https://doi.org/10.1007/978-3-030-58945-5_21.

18. Mofid MM, Teitelbaum S, Suissa D, et al. Report on mortality from gluteal fat grafting: recommendations from the ASERF task force. Aesthetic Surg J 2017; 37(7):796–806.

19. Singh D. Female judgment of male attractiveness and desirability for relationships: role of waist-to-hip ratio and financial status. J Pers Soc Psychol 1995;69(6):1089.

20. Singh D. Universal allure of the hourglass figure: an evolutionary theory of female physical attractiveness. Clin Plast Surg 2006;33:359370.

21. Manzaneda Cipriani RM, Adrianzen GA, Zulueta J, et al. Aesthetic preferences of the anterior thigh as a beauty factor in women. Plastic and Reconstructive Surgery - Global Open 2022;10(1):E4055.

22. Roberts TL, Weinfeld AB, Bruner TW, et al. "Universal" and ethnic ideals of beautiful buttocks are best obtained by autologous micro fat grafting and liposuction. Clin Plast Surg 2006;33(3):371–94.

23. Vartanian E, Gould DJ, Hammoudeh ZS, et al. The ideal thigh: a crowdsourcing-based assessment of ideal thigh aesthetic and implications for gluteal fat grafting. Aesthetic Surg J 2018;38(8):861–9.

24. Wong WW, Motakef S, Lin Y, et al. Redefining the ideal buttocks: a population analysis. Plast Reconstr Surg 2016;137(6):1739–47.

25. Durán Vega HC, Cardenas L. Chapter 19: Infiltraçao de gordura nos gluteos. In: Lipo de definicao 3a geracao da lipoaspiracao. Osvaldo Saldanha261, 1st edition. Editorial Di livros Editora; 2021. p. 272.

26. Cárdenas-Camarena L, Durán H. Improvement of the gluteal contour: modern concepts with systematized lipoinjection. Clin Plast Surg 2018; 45(2):237–47.

27. Durán Vega HC, de Baco F, Echaury AL. Vectorial treatment of infragluteal fold. Plastic and Reconstructive Surgery - Global Open 2023;11(Issue 1): E4750. Lippincott Williams and Wilkins.

28. Manzaneda Cipriani RM, Babaitis R, Vega HD, et al. Intramuscular posterior thigh volumization: an aesthetic and harmonious transition to the gluteal region (Hv-FAT). Plast Reconstr Surg Glob Open 2023; 11(4):e4918.

29. Durán H. The lipocontour technique. In: *Aesthetic surgery of the buttock*. Cham, Switzerland: Springer; 2023. p. 219–30. https://doi.org/10.1007/978-3-031-13802-7_15.

30. Presented by Dan del Vecchio and Pat Pazmiño, The Aesthetic Meeting 2022, San Diego Convention Center in San Diego Cal.USA.

31. Roberts TL, Toledo LS, Badin AZ. Augmentation of the buttocks by micro fat grafting. Aesthetic Surg J 2001;21(4):311–9.

32. Frojo G, Halani SH, Pessa JE, et al. Deep subcutaneous gluteal fat compartments: anatomy and clinical implications. Aesthetic Surg J 2023;43(1): 76–83.

33. Ramos-Gallardo G, Hernández MÁL, Cuenca-Pardo J, et al. Infection in the operated buttock. In: *Aesthetic surgery of the buttock*. Cham, Switzerland: Springer; 2023. p. 417–25. https://doi.org/10.1007/978-3-031-13802-7_29.

34. Ghavami A, Villanueva NL, Amirlak B. Gluteal ligamentous anatomy and its implication in safe buttock augmentation. Plast Reconstr Surg 2018;142(2): 363–71.

Ultrasound-Guided Gluteal Fat Grafting: A to Z

Pat Pazmiño, MD*

KEYWORDS

- Brazilian butt lift • BBL • Gluteal fat grafting • Buttock augmentation • Buttock enlargement
- Fat grafting • Ultrasound-Guided Fat Transfer

KEY POINTS

- Gluteal fat grafting has had unusually high complication and mortality rates when surgeons inadvertently injected fat graft into the muscles and intramuscular veins.
- Modern ultrasound probes combine low-cost ultrasound emitters, artificial intelligence, and wireless connectivity into an inexpensive, portable tool that can be readily used in the sterile environment of the operating room.
- Ultrasound allows surgeons to visualize and manipulate the anatomy of the subcutaneous region.
- Ultrasound allows surgeons to confirm that their fat graft is only placed subcutaneously.
- Ultrasound can create video to document the subcutaneous only placement of fat graft, protecting the patient and surgeon.

INTRODUCTION

Gluteal contouring and augmentation have become an extremely popular and powerful tools in body contouring surgery. This has been driven by patient demand as society's ideals of beauty have continued to expand. Beauty is now accepted at any size and in many shapes. Patients are specifically requesting smaller waists, fuller buttocks, and rounder hips.[1–4]

Surgeons have always been able to accentuate gluteal contours with abdominal and trunk fat extraction and liposuction alone. Small asymmetries and depressions can also be effectively corrected with liposhifting and equalization.[5–7] However, true gluteal augmentation can only be accomplished with solid silicone gluteal implants or fat grafting.

Gluteal fat grafting has been proven to be effective in the plastic surgery literature and, more recently, has been memorialized by patients and surgeons throughout social media.[2,8] This is a powerful surgery but it is safe, and effective execution is technique dependent.

During the last 11 years, there has been an extraordinarily high number of complications and mortalities after gluteal fat grafting. Deaths after gluteal fat grafting have occurred due to severe anemia, sepsis, and abdominal organ perforations but the most common fatal complication remains pulmonary fat embolism (PFE).[9] A 2-hit hypothesis for PFE notes that 2 factors must be present: (1) intramuscular fat graft and (2) a gluteal venous injury. When intramuscular fat grafting is performed, the cannula can injure intramuscular gluteal veins and nearby fat graft can enter these injured veins.[3,10–12] The now intravascular fat graft travels to the heart, lungs, and brain with fatal results.

MRI venogram studies have demonstrated that the gluteal muscles have a dense, irregular, and asymmetric plexus of large intramuscular gluteal veins.[13] Therefore, it is not enough to avoid the main trunks of the inferior and superior gluteal veins. The entire unpredictable intramuscular venous tree must be avoided. By performing only subcutaneous gluteal fat grafting, the intramuscular gluteal veins can be avoided, and pulmonary

Division of Plastic Surgery, University of Miami
* 848 Brickell Avenue, Suite 820 Miami, FL 33131.
E-mail address: cps@miamia.com

Clin Plastic Surg 50 (2023) 587–601
https://doi.org/10.1016/j.cps.2023.07.002

fat emboli can be prevented. Until recently, surgeons could only perform gluteal fat grafting as a blind procedure, only with palpation.

It is because of the possible dangers with this procedure that plastic surgeons must not abandon gluteal fat grafting. Gluteal fat grafting is a powerful tool that can augment tissue, correct deformities, and create impressive results that cannot be produced any other way. Because of this, high patient demand for this procedure will continue. If board-certified plastic surgeons stop performing this procedure, interested patients will simply go to the non–board-certified practitioners and even more deaths will occur. As researchers and patient advocates, plastic surgeons must study this technique and determine how gluteal fat grafting can be performed safely and consistently.

EPIDEMIOLOGY

Deaths from fat pulmonary emboli have occurred throughout the world but in the United States, South Florida has been the epicenter of these tragedies. In the last 13 years, in South Florida alone, 25 deaths from fat pulmonary emboli have been identified.[9,14] The author observed 11 autopsies performed by the Miami Dade County Medical Examiner. The postmortem results noted that intramuscular fat graft was present in every autopsy.

In 2017, the Multi-Society Task Force for Safety in Gluteal Fat Grafting (Rubin, Mills, Saltz, and colleagues) designed cadaver studies to further understand the mechanics of a PFE. The Task Force invited leading gluteal surgeons to perform gluteal fat grafting with dyed lipoaspirate under fluoroscopy. After the injection, the specimens received expert dissections to demonstrate the placement of the fat graft. The Task Force measured safer cannula angles and lengths to avoid gluteal vein trunk injuries. In 2018, the Task Force issued guidelines for safe gluteal fat injection, which included constant vigilance of the cannula tip during fat grafting, a rigid cannula system, and most importantly to avoid intramuscular fat injection by staying above the deep gluteal fascia on the superior surface of the gluteus maximus at all times.[15,16]

Therefore, by the end of 2018, plastic surgeons understood the importance of avoiding intramuscular fat graft injections. An international survey of plastic surgeons in early 2019 noted that the standard of care in gluteal fat grafting had changed in that 85.5% of surgeons were injecting only in the subcutaneous space.[17] In June of 2019, the state of Florida acknowledged this new standard of care by mandating that all gluteal fat grafting be performed in the subcutaneous space, and that surgeons who injected fat under the deep gluteal fascia could lose their medical license. Yet, despite these cadaver studies, autopsy findings, society recommendations, and Florida Board of Medicine mandates, deaths from pulmonary fat emboli continued to increase in South Florida.[14]

The South Florida surgeons who had a pulmonary fat emboli death used different fat graft volumes, different patient positions, different access incisions, and different cannula styles. The one factor that all of these deaths had in common was that every surgeon insisted that they were subcutaneous and above the deep gluteal fascia at all times. Unfortunately, the autopsies disagreed. The South Florida experience demonstrates that surgeons currently do not have a consistent and reliable way to always know the position of their cannula tip during gluteal fat grafting. Moreover, surgeons have no way to prove that they only injected fat subcutaneously and to document that they never injected fat into the gluteal muscles to protect themselves for medicolegal reasons.

GLUTEAL FAT GRAFTING SAFETY GAP

The inability of surgeons to consistently visualize in real time the tip of their cannula and confirm subcutaneous only fat graft placement was the safety gap that prevented consistently safe gluteal fat grafting. Ultrasound can help fill this safety gap. In the last 2 years, ultrasound equipment has become portable, wireless, and affordable allowing for its use in the sterile field of the operating room (OR). For the first time, surgeons can now use ultrasound technology to visualize the position of their cannula in the subcutaneous space during fat graft injection and document the safe execution of this procedure with sonographic video. Ultrasound visualization can be used with any cannula style or injection system.[18] Real-time intraoperative ultrasound visualization can help the surgeon perform fat harvesting and accurate fat grafting into the unique spaces of the subcutaneous region.[19] This will not only make for a safer surgeon but a better surgeon—a surgeon who can manipulate subcutaneous anatomy not appreciable without ultrasound.

ULTRASOUND PHYSICS AND EQUIPMENT

Ultrasound waves are mechanical sound waves with a frequency above the human range of hearing (>20 kHz), thus *ultra* sound. The higher the frequency of an ultrasound probe, the better resolution but the lesser the frequency, deeper the ultrasound can penetrate tissue. Ultrasound probes with a low frequency (<10 MHz) can visualize deep body structures, whereas ultrasound probes with a high frequency can visualize superficial structures. Clinical diagnostic ultrasound ranges from 1 to 20 MHz. Obstetricians use ultrasounds in the range of 2.5 MHz to visualize deep abdominal organs. Vascular surgeons assess deep arteries and veins with 5 MHz machines, and breast surgeons visualize breast tissue with 10-MHz ultrasound probes. Dermatologists use ultrasound probes of 20 MHz to visualize the skin and superficial adnexa. As plastic surgeons are most concerned with subcutaneous structures, ultrasound probes of 11 to 20 MHz are most appropriate.[20]

Traditional ultrasound machines used the piezoelectric effect by alternating voltage across a quartz crystal. This created fluctuations in pressure across the crystal and then ultimately produced sound waves. Traditional ultrasound machines were thus delicate and expensive. Recently, ultrasound probes using microcrystals or microchips to produce the ultrasound waves have become commercially available. These units couple this technology with artificial intelligence to optimize the image quality and wireless connectivity to create a small portable unit that can conveniently be used by surgeons in the sterile environment of the operating room.

During the past 9 years, the author has used 7 different ultrasound systems for gluteal fat grafting. Due to their small form factor, 1 of 2 portable systems is being used for real-time intraoperative ultrasound: the Clarius L7 HD3 (Clarius Mobile Health, Vancouver, Canada, US $3,400) or the Butterfly iQ (Butterfly Imaging, US $2,000 with US $420 annual subscription) (**Fig. 1**). The Clarius L7 HD3 is a 4 to 13-Mhz high-frequency linear portable, waterproof, wireless ultrasound probe (maximum depth of 11 cm) that can be placed entirely in a sterile probe cover and can stream a high-resolution ultrasound video to Apple iOS or Android tablets. Both systems will upload their data to the cloud so that ultrasound still images and video can be accessed on a computer or added to a patient chart. The Butterfly iQ+ (Butterfly Imaging, US $4,499) ultrasound probe uses microchips, rather than piezoelectric quartz crystals to generate the ultrasound waves. The Butterfly iQ+ is a medium-resolution probe with a range of 1 to 10 MHz and a maximum scan depth of 30 cm. The Butterfly iQ + connects to a smart phone or tablet with a cable necessitating a longer probe cover for a tethered connection in the operating room suite (see **Fig. 1**; **Fig. 2**).

It is important to note that any ultrasound probe can be used with any injection technique or

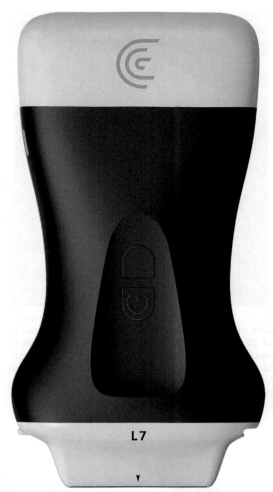

Fig. 1. The Clarius L7 HD3 ultrasound probe is a 4 to 13 MHz high-frequency linear L7 HD3 portable, waterproof, wireless ultrasound probe (maximum depth of 11 cm) that can be placed entirely in a sterile probe cover and can stream a high-resolution ultrasound video to Apple iOS or Android tablets. (L7 HD3, Linear Scanner. With permission from © Clarius 2022.)

instrumentation. Surgeons interested in trying ultrasound-guided gluteal fat grafting can simply borrow an ultrasound probe from their hospital, surgery center, emergency room, or anesthesia provider for their first cases.

GLUTEAL ANATOMY AND ULTRASOUND

The pelvic bony framework, gluteal muscles, gluteal fat, and skin have been well described in the surgical and radiologic literature.[21] Ultrasound can help us understand and then manipulate the subcutaneous zone. Cadaver dissections have actually identified 2 gluteal fasciae (**Fig. 3**).

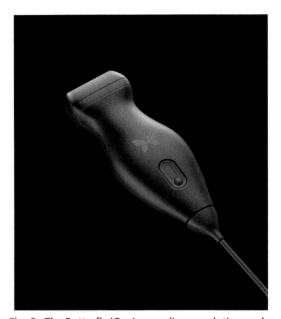

Fig. 2. The Butterfly iQ+ is a medium resolution probe with a range of 1 to 10 MHz and a maximum scan depth of 30 cm. The Butterfly iQ connects to an Android or Apple iOS smart phone or tablet with a cable necessitating a longer probe cover for a tethered connection in the operating room suite. (Butterfly iQ+. With permission from © 2023 Butterfly Network, Inc.)

The deep gluteal fascia is adhered to the external surface of the gluteus maximus muscle. This is the fascial plane that the Multi Society Task Force has recommended surgeons to never place fat graft underneath.[10,15]

However, there also exists a second fascia layer (the superficial gluteal fascia) within the subcutaneous zone above the deep gluteal fascia and below the dermis. The superficial gluteal fascia is thinner than the deep gluteal fascia and like "bubble wrap" in that the fused fascia lamellae irregularly separate and are impregnated with fat lobules. This superficial gluteal fascia can only be appreciated in an open dissection or with ultrasound visualization. The superficial gluteal fascia divides the subcutaneous region into 2 spaces: the superficial subcutaneous space under the dermis and above the superficial gluteal fascia, and the deep subcutaneous space under the superficial gluteal fascia and above the deep gluteal fascia.

The superficial gluteal fascia is analogous to Scarpa fascia in the abdomen and divides the subcutaneous zone into 2 subcutaneous spaces: the superficial subcutaneous space (between the dermis and the superficial gluteal fascia) and the deep subcutaneous space (between the superficial gluteal fascia and the deep gluteal fascia)[22] (**Fig. 4**).

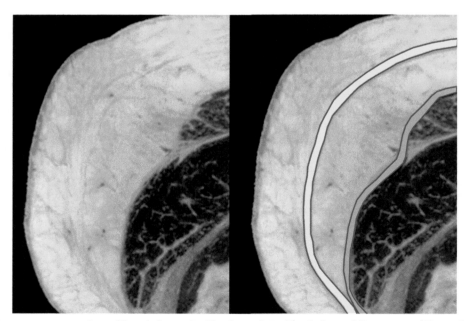

Fig. 3. Transverse cross section of female buttocks. The deep gluteal fascia (green) lies on top of the surface of the gluteus maximus muscle. The superficial gluteal fascia (yellow) is above the deep gluteal fascia and below the dermis and divides the subcutaneous region into 2 spaces. (*From* Pazmiño, P. (2020). ultraBBL: Brazilian Butt Lift Using Real-Time Intraoperative Ultrasound Guidance. In: Garcia Jr., O. (eds) Ultrasound-Assisted Liposuction. Springer, Cham. https://doi.org/10.1007/978-3-030-26875-6_10.)

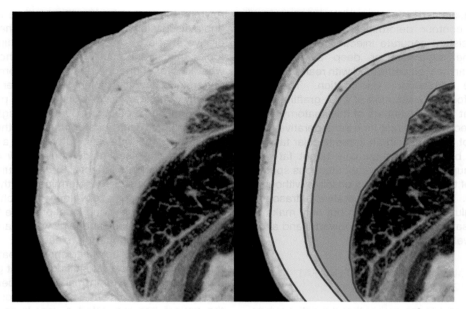

Fig. 4. Transverse cross section of female buttocks. The superficial gluteal fascia divides the subcutaneous region into 2 spaces. The superficial subcutaneous space (yellow) is below the skin and above the superficial gluteal fascia. The deep subcutaneous space (green) is below the superficial gluteal fascia and above the deep gluteal fascia. Ultrasound allows the surgeon to accurately enter each space and manipulate it while always remaining above the deep gluteal fascia. (*From* Pazmiño, P. (2020). ultraBBL: Brazilian Butt Lift Using Real-Time Intraoperative Ultrasound Guidance. In: Garcia Jr., O. (eds) Ultrasound-Assisted Liposuction. Springer, Cham. https://doi.org/10.1007/978-3-030-26875-6_10.)

DEEP GLUTEAL FASCIA: SAFETY

The dynamic cadaver studies of Del Vecchio and colleagues emphasized the importance of the deep gluteal fascia in performing safe gluteal fat grafting.[23] These cadaver studies showed that if fat graft was placed above an intact deep gluteal fascia, the deep fascia would act as a "stout wall" and prevent fat graft from entering the gluteus maximus or the intramuscular veins that act as the entry point to fat emboli. Del Vecchio and colleagues also demonstrated that deep gluteal fascia with less than 1 cm fenestrations could still prevent the migration of fat graft into the muscle but that deep gluteal fascia with defects larger than 1 cm would allow subcutaneously placed fat graft to migrate through the deep gluteal fascia and enter the muscle belly and veins. These findings should provide great comfort for gluteal surgeons because if fat graft is consistently placed above the deep gluteal fascia, the patient will be protected from pulmonary fat emboli. Furthermore, if the gluteal surgeon inadvertently pierces the deep gluteal fascia with the grafting cannula, this will not make a defect large than 1 cm and the patient will still be protected from pulmonary fat emboli. Therefore, to perform safe gluteal fat grafting, the surgeon must consistently place the fat graft above the deep gluteal fascia.

SUPERFICIAL GLUTEAL FASCIA: PRECISION

Similar to the superficial musculoaponeurotic system (SMAS) for facial surgeons, gluteal surgeons can identify and manipulate the superficial gluteal fascia to improve their surgical results. For the first time, ultrasound allows surgeons to target the superficial subcutaneous space or the deep subcutaneous space with millimeter accuracy, always staying above the deep gluteal fascia.

Cadaver studies have examined the deep and superficial subcutaneous spaces and noted that they are markedly different. The superficial subcutaneous space has a dense highly organized fibroseptal network, whereas the deep subcutaneous space does not have this dense fibroseptal network but rather is organized into distinct compartments.[24] This differential anatomy is visible in cross sections of this area (see Fig 3). This differential anatomy also has important clinical effects.

If the superficial gluteal fascia remains intact, it can retain the fat graft that is specifically injected below it, like the casing of a sausage. Fat graft injected into the deep subcutaneous space (above the deep gluteal fascia and below the superficial gluteal fascia) can create excellent volume and central dome projection, similar to a subfascial implant. Fat graft precisely injected into the superficial subcutaneous space (above the superficial gluteal fascia and below the skin) can correct superficial contour deformities and depressions. The consistent accurate injection of fat graft to either the superficial or deep subcutaneous spaces can only be performed with real-time intraoperative ultrasound visualization. This has allowed for the description of a fat grafting technique that takes advantage of this anatomy.[19]

A surgeon can use real-time intraoperative ultrasound not only to avoid an intramuscular fat graft injection but also to accurately target fat graft into the superficial or deep subcutaneous spaces. Neither of these techniques is possible without ultrasound. Real-time intraoperative ultrasound-guided gluteal fat grafting can not only make fat grafting safer but much more powerful and accurate as well.

ULTRASOUND-GUIDED GLUTEAL FAT GRAFTING: TECHNIQUE

It is important to remember that the entire subcutaneous zone (including both the superficial and deep gluteal spaces) ranges in thickness from 1 cm (outer hips) to 3 to 4 cm (central gluteal dome). This means that gluteal surgeons must graft in a thin space under a curving dome of varying thickness. This small variable target may account for the inadvertent deep intramuscular injections by well-intentioned surgeons grafting without ultrasound visualization.

Real-time intraoperative ultrasound can actually be used with any cannula or liposuction/fat grafting system. However, when a syringe fat grafting system is used, both of the surgeon's hands are occupied. One hand must hold the syringe while the other hand pushes the plunger to inject the fat. In this scenario, the surgical assistant or scrub tech must control the sterile ultrasound probe, making coordination with the injecting surgeon difficult. To allow the surgeon to control the fat grafting system and the ultrasound probe simultaneously, a power-assisted liposuction system (PAL, MicroAire Charlottesville, VA) is used in conjunction with a peristaltic pump for controlled propulsion of the fat graft. In this manner, the surgeon can inject fat via expansion vibration lipofilling (EVL) with one hand and control the ultrasound probe with the nondominant hand.[25]

PREOPERATIVE ASSESSMENT

Similar to all plastic surgery, careful preoperative assessment and planning before gluteal contouring and fat grafting is essential. The surgeon should sit with the patient to understand their goals, priorities, and areas of importance.

Asymmetries must be identified before surgery, and a discussion should be held about the preoperative shape of the patient's waist, hips, buttocks, thighs, and back. The surgeon should ask what kind of shape the patient would prefer and understand how the patient would prefer to specifically change their waist, hips, point of maximum hip projection, buttocks, thighs, and back. Within each anatomic zone, the bony framework, the muscles, fatty layer, and skin should be assessed to determine how each of these components affects the contour. Ultrasound can be used to determine the thickness of the subcutaneous envelope in each region and plan the quantity and location of the fat graft in each subcutaneous space as well as any areas of adhesion that should be released.

Digital imaging is helpful to show the patient the effects of liposuction, fat shifting, and fat grafting. It is even more useful in managing expectations and showing the patient what is not possible. If the patient has requested a very large volume result, digital imaging can illustrate what is reasonable and safe and open a discussion on staging the procedure. Patients interested in large volume results that would be best served with staged procedures can be shown where fat can be left undisturbed and ready for harvest in a second round of fat harvest and grafting.

Once the final operative plan has been decided, the surgeon should discuss the recovery, expected fat resorption rates, and limitations on postoperative activity.

SURGICAL EQUIPMENT AND SET UP
Fat Trap Canister

It is preferable that the fat graft remain in a liquid state for smooth propulsion through our EVL system. When harvesting fat, a vacuum is established through the tubing and any aspirated fat is captured within the canister. Many canister models are available and have been tried but the simplest one is preferred—a reusable plastic canister with a lid and no openings or spigots at the bottom. For a fat grafting procedure using EVL and the MicroAire system, 2 different types of liposuction tubing are necessary. Standard liposuction tubing (both ends with large openings) (PSI-TEC Tubing, Ref PT-5558, Mentor, Irving, TX) is used to connect the suction source to the canister lid. MicroAire tapered tubing (Ref PAL-1200, MicroAire, Charlottesville, VA) is then used to connect the other port on the canister lid to the MicroAire liposuction cannula. The lipoaspirate that is collected is allowed to separate with gravity and time to allow the fat to separate from the tumescent fluid. Openings or spigots at the bottom of the fat trap canisters act as chokepoints in the fat grafting system during EVL.

PERISTALTIC PUMP FOR FAT GRAFTING

A peristaltic pump system is used for infiltration of the tumescent fluid and for controlled fat grafting via EVL, as well.

Surgical Technique

Liposuction of the torso and fat grafting to the gluteal areas and hips is designed to be an outpatient procedure performed under general anesthesia. Specific types of anesthesia do not effectively protect the patient from fatal complications such as pulmonary fat emboli. What does protect the patient is ensuring that there is no intramuscular fat injection. Ultrasound visualization can continuously confirm the real-time position of the cannula tip and keep the patient safe. Ultrasound-guided gluteal fat grafting is performed under general anesthesia to facilitate comfortable controlled extraction of deep and superficial fat and for maintenance of the airway when the patient is in the prone position.

LIPOSUCTION AND LIPOSCULPTURE

Surgeons often struggle with identifying the endpoint in liposuction. Some surgeons record the volume removed from one side and match this to the contralateral side. Other surgeons count the minutes of liposuction or ultrasound-assisted liposuction in one treatment area and match it to the contralateral side. We must keep in mind that ultimately, liposuction is sculpture. A sculptor does not weigh the amount of stone removed from one side and continues to chisel the opposite side until the same amount of stone has been removed. Similar to all sculpture, our liposuction surgical endpoint must be anatomic and symmetric. The anatomic endpoint of liposuction should be to achieve an esthetic symmetric result with flaps of consistent thickness throughout the torso. This process begins before surgery when the skin and fat thickness in all treatment areas are assessed, and asymmetries are highlighted. A strategy should be in place to differentially remove fat until the flap has a consistent thickness.

The incisions used for liposuction and fat grafting of the torso are designed to access all treatment areas and are placed in inconspicuous locations. On the anterior abdomen, one incision is placed inside the umbilicus at the 12 o'clock position. An incision in each inguinal crease is also made to access the anterior abdomen, lateral

abdomen, and waist and thighs. Posteriorly, 2 supragluteal incisions, 2 infragluteal incisions, and 1 intergluteal incision can be used (Fig. 5).

Once the patient is prepped and draped, 3 access incisions are made in the anterior abdomen—1 inside and at the bottom of the umbilicus and 2 inguinal incisions, each just under the bikini line. Skin protectors are placed within each incision to minimize abrasions and skin trauma. Tumescent fluid consisting of 1 L of normal saline and 1 ampoule of epinephrine (final epinephrine concentration of 1:1,000,000) is warmed and used in all treatment areas. A typical gluteal fat grafting case uses approximately 4000 to 5000 cc of tumescent fluid. Tumescent fluid is infiltrated into the treatment areas using the simultaneous separation and tumescence technique via the MicroAire system using a 3 mm exploded

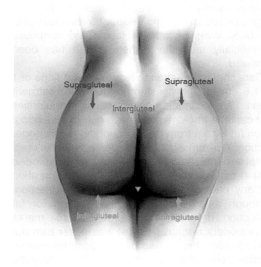

Fig. 5. Posterior gluteal access incisions: the supragluteal incisions are used for fat harvest of the back, waist, hips, flanks, and sides as well as fat grafting to the central dome and superior outer hip. The intergluteal incision is used for fat harvest of the back, along the lower latissimus dorsi, and for contouring the superior buttock as well as fat grafting to the dome and the supragluteal region. The infragluteal incisions are used for fat harvest, fat shifting, and fat grafting to the outer hips and thighs. (*From* Pazmiño, P. (2020). ultraBBL: Brazilian Butt Lift Using Real-Time Intraoperative Ultrasound Guidance. In: Garcia Jr., O. (eds) Ultrasound-Assisted Liposuction. Springer, Cham. https://doi.org/10.1007/978-3-030-26875-6_10.)

basket cannula.[26] As Del Vecchio and Wall described, this allows for the separation of subcutaneous tissue and a more rapid onset of the epinephrine vasoconstriction.

More importantly, fat separation before fat harvest, as described by Wall, is the crucial concept in body contouring.[7] When performing body sculpting, deformities are only created under suction. A deformity cannot occur when fat is displaced or separated without suction. For this reason, it is recommended to separate the fat as much as possible before fat harvest. Fat separation with a 5-mm exploded basket cannula after the infiltration of tumescent fluid and before fat extraction with suction allows the epinephrine to continue working, releases fibers and adhesions, allows for easy subsequent extraction, and creates small fat grafts that can fill and correct small local irregularities. Fat separation continues until the cannula can move through the treatment area without resistance. No suction has been applied up to this point. Once the separation phase has been completed, fat extraction under suction can begin. Extraction begins deep, at a level just over the deep investing muscle fascia and continues superficially until the esthetic result has been achieved.

Care should be taken to leave skin-fat flaps of 1 to 1.5 cm in thickness throughout all treatment areas. Large cannulas do not cause irregularities and cannula track marks. These deformities occur when fat is torn from the surrounding tissue under suction. A 5-mm exploded basket cannula is used for fat separation and fat harvest. A large exploded basket cannula works very well for fat separation but any cannula can be used for fat extraction. Although a large cannula can be used for fat extraction, deformities and cannula track marks do not occur because the fat was never torn out with suction—the fat had been separated without suction during the separation phase and only the loose fat was removed with suction.

To create a uniform thickness of this skin-fat flap circumferentially around the torso, we begin by establishing this thickness first on one side of the patient's waist and flanks and then matching this thickness on the contralateral side, and finally throughout the anterior abdomen and throughout the back. Therefore, every procedure begins with the patient in the lateral decubitus position because this allows for inferior displacement of the abdominal contents and access to the deep fat of the waist, flanks, lower back, as well as the left costal margin and the left lateral anterior abdomen.

The procedure begins with the patient in the right lateral decubitus (left side up) position. The supragluteal and intergluteal incisions are used to access the left outer thigh, hips, waist, flank, lower back, costal margin, and lateral anterior abdomen. Once these areas have been tumesced and the subcutaneous tissue has been separated without suction, the fat is then harvested under suction. Once the left side has been completed, the patient is then placed into the left lateral decubitus (right side up) position and the right outer thigh, hip, waist, flank, lower back, right costal margin, and the right lateral anterior abdomen are tumesced, receive fat separation without suction, and finally, the loosened fat is extracted with suction. This continues until the skin-fat flap thickness on this side matches the contralateral side. At this time, the patient is returned to the supine position and the anterior abdomen is treated until the thickness of the skin-fat flap of the anterior abdomen matches the sides. If the patient requested liposculpture or abdominal etching, it is performed at this time. The inner thighs can be addressed in the supine position, as well. When all fat extraction has been completed, drains are placed through the inguinal incisions, sutured securely, and the patient is placed in the prone position. Once the patient is in the prone position, we check the peak inspiratory pressure and if a marked increase is noted compared with its supine value, chest rolls may be placed longitudinally along the lateral chest. In our experience, this is necessary in less than 1% of cases. The prone position is ideal to treat the bilateral lateral back, lower back, sacral area, and supragluteal contour. All areas will be tumesced, receive fat separation without suction, and loose fat removal under suction until the skin-fat flap thickness has been reached and our planned anatomic contours have been achieved. The patient is now ready for real-time intraoperative ultrasound-guided fat grafting.

FAT GRAFTING USING THE EXPANSION VIBRATION LIPOFILLING

The Multi-Society Task Force for Safety in Gluteal Fat Grafting recommended a rigid cannula greater than 3 mm in diameter to avoid inadvertent arcing or bending of the cannula because it is pushed through the gluteal tissue. They also warn of the bending at the Luer interface of many cannulas and recommend a more rigid system.[7,27] More importantly, if the surgeon uses one hand to hold the body of a syringe and the other hand to push the syringe plunger during injection, the surgeon does not have a free hand to palpate the tip of the cannula during fat grafting. For these 3 important reasons, the author recommends using a PAL system (MicroAire Charlottesville, VA) paired with a peristaltic pump to propel the fat graft during injection, better described as EVL.[25] To allow for smooth, controlled propulsion of the fat graft through the tubing system, the fat graft should be liquid. After fat harvest, the lipoaspirate is allowed to settle via gravity and the bottom aqueous portion is extracted, leaving a still fluid lipoaspirate for fat grafting.

A wide variety of cannulas can be used for fat grafting. The author prefers a "candy cane" cannula (Helix Tri-Port III, MicroAire) because the multiple openings avoid the single-hole obstruction of other cannulas and having all openings on one surface allow for precise directional fat grafting in the subcutaneous space(Fig. 6).

Fat grafting is performed under real-time intraoperative ultrasound guidance through the intergluteal and supragluteal access incisions. The infragluteal access incision is only used for addressing the outer thighs and hips.

REAL-TIME INTRAOPERATIVE ULTRASOUND VISUALIZATION OF FAT GRAFTING

All gluteal preoperative markings are reinforced including the horizontal line marking the point of greatest hip projection (at a level bisecting the intergluteal crease), as well as other areas that will require volume, adhesion release, correction of asymmetries, and so forth.

An Android or iOS tablet is mounted on an IV pole facing the gluteal area and the surgeon. The portable wireless ultrasound probe and a Bluetooth computer mouse are placed into a sterile probe cover (6″ × 48″ Soft Flex Probe Cover REF 20-PC648 Advance Medical Designs Marietta, GA) and brought onto the field. The ultrasound probe is placed on the skin over the first treatment area (central mound) and the sterile computer mouse is used to adjust the ultrasound probe's depth of field, gain, mode, and contrast. Recording of the ultrasound-guided fat grafting procedure begins.

The surgeon will hold the MicroAire handle and cannula with the dominant hand, the ultrasound probe with the nondominant hand to visualize the

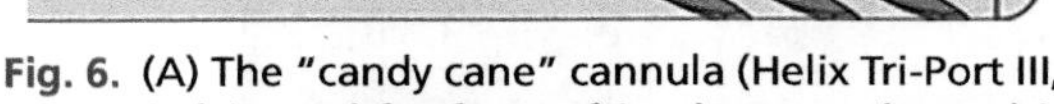

Fig. 6. (A) The "candy cane" cannula (Helix Tri-Port III, MicroAire) is used for fat grafting because the multiple openings avoid clogging by the fat graft and having all openings on only one side of the cannula allows for precise directional fat grafting. (*From* Pazmiño, P. (2020). ultraBBL: Brazilian Butt Lift Using Real-Time Intraoperative Ultrasound Guidance. In: Garcia Jr., O. (eds) Ultrasound-Assisted Liposuction. Springer, Cham. https://doi.org/10.1007/978-3-030-26875-6_10.)

cannula tip and control the propulsion of the aqueous fat graft with a foot pedal.

The order of gluteal fat grafting begins centrally to establish projection over the central gluteal dome, then laterally to the hips, and finally into the supragluteal and medial gluteal regions. The cannula is inserted through the supragluteal or intergluteal incisions and advanced into the treatment zone until it is visualized by the ultrasound. To create a significant central dome projection, the cannula tip is placed with ultrasound guidance into the deep subcutaneous space (under the superficial gluteal fascia and above the deep gluteal fascia) and fat graft is precisely injected. The cannula tip is always visualized and care is taken never to place the cannula tip below the deep gluteal fascia because this would result in an intramuscular injection. Any adhesions within the deep subcutaneous space can be visualized and released allowing for even distribution of the fat graft throughout this zone. To correct superficial skin depressions and asymmetries, the superficial subcutaneous space (above the superficial gluteal fascia and below the skin) is specifically addressed. Ultrasound-guided fat separation and release of adhesions is first performed in the superficial subcutaneous space followed by controlled fat injection. Care is taken to keep the superficial gluteal fascia intact because this will maintain separate deep and superficial subcutaneous spaces and prevent blowout irregularities. In this manner, the 2 anatomic subcutaneous spaces can be individually addressed in each anatomic area (Figs. 7–9).

Real-time intraoperative ultrasound-guided fat grafting allows the surgeon to consistently avoid penetrating the deep gluteal fascia and prevent an inadvertent intramuscular fat graft injection. It also lets the surgeon accurately manipulate the structures of the subcutaneous region and to precisely fat graft into the deep or superficial subcutaneous spaces. Ultrasound video of the entire fat grafting process can easily be created to serve as definitive documentation that at no time was there an intramuscular injection. Real-time intraoperative ultrasound allows for precise fat grafting into the subcutaneous spaces and can keep the patient and the surgeon safe.

PATIENT CASES
Case One

A 42-year-old G1P1 Hispanic woman presents with lipodystrophy of the abdomen, waist, sides, flanks, and thighs and loss of volume, asymmetry and ptosis of the gluteal areas and hips, bilaterally. The patient stated that she would prefer the

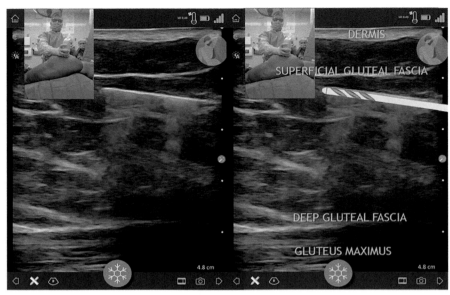

Fig. 7. Central dome with fat grafting cannula in deep gluteal space: The "candy cane" fat grafting cannula is directly beneath the superficial gluteal fascia and is facing inferiorly. It is displacing the superficial gluteal fascia superiorly to allow for expansion of the deep gluteal space. The deep gluteal fascia and the gluteus maximus are noted to be 4 cm below the skin surface. (*From* Pazmiño, P. (2020). ultraBBL: Brazilian Butt Lift Using Real-Time Intraoperative Ultrasound Guidance. In: Garcia Jr., O. (eds) Ultrasound-Assisted Liposuction. Springer, Cham. https://doi.org/10.1007/978-3-030-26875-6_10.)

lipodystrophy of her abdomen and back correct, as well as a rounder and fuller gluteal contour. The patient was evaluated on physical examination, and it was noted that she had significant lipodystrophy of the anterior abdomen, waist, flanks, lower back, and sacral area as well as depressions and volume loss of the outer hips and gluteal ptosis.

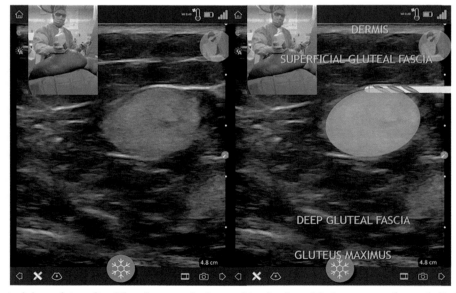

Fig. 8. Central dome fat graft exiting the cannula. Fat grafting begins with the aqueous fat graft (light gray hypoechoic bubble) leaving the inferior surface of the "candy cane" cannula under the superficial gluteal fascia and within the deep subcutaneous space. (*From* Pazmiño, P. (2020). ultraBBL: Brazilian Butt Lift Using Real-Time Intraoperative Ultrasound Guidance. In: Garcia Jr., O. (eds) Ultrasound-Assisted Liposuction. Springer, Cham. https://doi.org/10.1007/978-3-030-26875-6_10.)

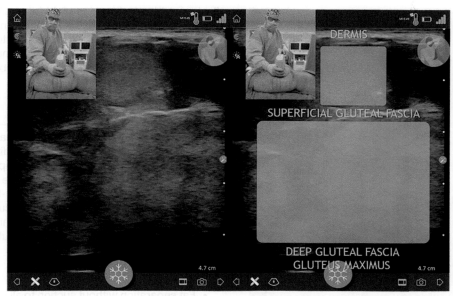

Fig. 9. Outer hips, after fat grafting to both spaces. Fat graft has expanded the superficial subcutaneous space and the deep subcutaneous space. This is essential when filling the outer hips. (*From* Pazmiño, P. (2020). ultraBBL: Brazilian Butt Lift Using Real-Time Intraoperative Ultrasound Guidance. In: Garcia Jr., O. (eds) Ultrasound-Assisted Liposuction. Springer, Cham. https://doi.org/10.1007/978-3-030-26875-6_10.)

Patient's Priorities

The patient stated that she would prefer to extract as much fat from the anterior abdomen, waist, and flanks as possible. She also stated that she would prefer a low waist-to-hip ratio (less than 0.6) and would prefer to fill the lateral gluteal hollows.

Operative Challenges

Fibrous tissue of the back and sacral area may make fat separation and extraction difficult in these important anatomic areas. Outer hip contour after fat grafting will rely on survival of the fat graft, making achieving the desired waist-to-hip ratio with outer hip fat grafting alone, difficult.

Surgical Plan

- Fat separation without suction to all areas, followed by fat extraction under suction.
- Deep space fat grafting to the central domes, supragluteal area, and outer hips at the point of greatest projection.
- Superficial space fat grafting to correct superficial concavities at the outer hips.
- To more reliably achieve the patient's desired waist-to-hip ratio, extract as much fat throughout the waist and flanks as possible, rather than rely on the survival of fat graft in the outer hips (**Fig. 10**).

RESULT

The patient received ultrasound-guided gluteal fat grafting with fat separation and fat extraction of the abdomen, waist, flanks, lower back, and sacral areas. She received 900 cc of ultrasound-guided fat graft per side. A total of 700 cc of fat graft was placed in the deep subcutaneous space (above the deep gluteal fascia and below the superficial gluteal fascia) for the creation of gluteal volume, central dome projection, and outer hip expansion. She then received 200 cc of fat graft to the superficial subcutaneous space (above the superficial gluteal fascia and below the skin) to the outer hips, bilaterally. The patient is shown with a 6-month result and is satisfied with the result (**Figs. 11** and **12**).

Case Two

A 27-year-old G0P0 African American woman presents with lipodystrophy of the abdomen, waist, sides, flanks, and thighs and loss of volume, asymmetry and ptosis of the gluteal areas and hips, bilaterally. The patient was evaluated on physical examination, and it was noted that she had significant lipodystrophy of the anterior abdomen, waist, flanks, lower back, and sacral area as well as volume loss of the outer hips and gluteal ptosis.

Patient's Priorities

The patient stated she would prefer to extract as much fat as possible from the abdomen, waist,

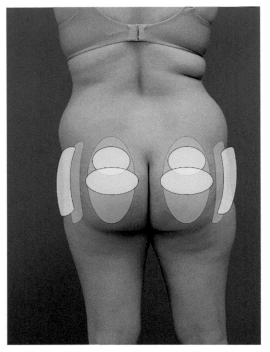

Fig. 10. UltraBBL Case 1: ultrasound-guided fat grafting plan. Gluteal fat grafting was planned to the deep subcutaneous spaces (green) to increase projection and add volume. Fat grafting to the superficial subcutaneous spaces (yellow) would supplement the deep volume and correct superficial irregularities. (*From* Pazmiño, P. (2020). ultraBBL: Brazilian Butt Lift Using Real-Time Intraoperative Ultrasound Guidance. In: Garcia Jr., O. (eds) Ultrasound-Assisted Liposuction. Springer, Cham. https://doi.org/10.1007/978-3-030-26875-6_10.)

flanks, and back. She also stated that she would prefer to maximize her gluteal volume and create a spherical contour. The patient requested a low hip-to-waist ratio (less than 0.6) and a high point of maximum hip projection (2 cm above the midpoint of the intergluteal cleft).

Operative Challenges

Fibrous tissue of the back and sacral area may make fat separation and extraction difficult in these important anatomic areas. Outer hip contour after fat grafting will rely on survival of the fat graft, making achieving the desired waist-to-hip ratio with outer hip fat grafting alone, difficult. More fibrous tissue superiorly along the outer hip makes a high point of maximal projection difficult.

SURGICAL PLAN

- Fat separation without suction to all areas, followed by fat extraction under suction.
- Deep space fat grafting to the central domes, supragluteal area, and outer hips at a high point of greatest hip projection.
- Anticipate for additional adhesion release in both spaces along the outer hip before and after fat grafting for smooth graft distribution.
- Superficial space fat grafting to correct superficial concavities at the outer hips.
- To more reliably achieve the patient's desired waist-to-hip ratio, extract as much fat as possible throughout the waist and flanks, rather than rely on the survival of fat graft in the outer hips (**Fig. 13**).

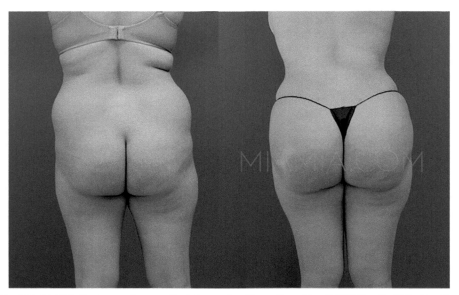

Fig. 11. UltraBBL CASE 1. Postoperative result at 6 months. (*From* Pazmiño, P. (2020). ultraBBL: Brazilian Butt Lift Using Real-Time Intraoperative Ultrasound Guidance. In: Garcia Jr., O. (eds) Ultrasound-Assisted Liposuction. Springer, Cham. https://doi.org/10.1007/978-3-030-26875-6_10.)

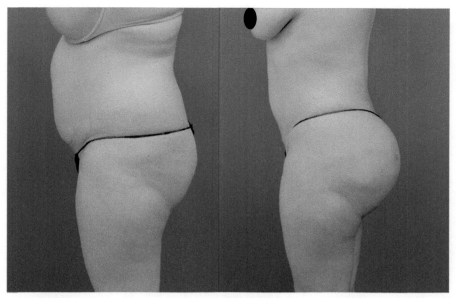

Fig. 12. UltraBBL CASE 1. Postoperative result at 6 months. (*From* Pazmiño, P. (2020). ultraBBL: Brazilian Butt Lift Using Real-Time Intraoperative Ultrasound Guidance. In: Garcia Jr., O. (eds) Ultrasound-Assisted Liposuction. Springer, Cham. https://doi.org/10.1007/978-3-030-26875-6_10.)

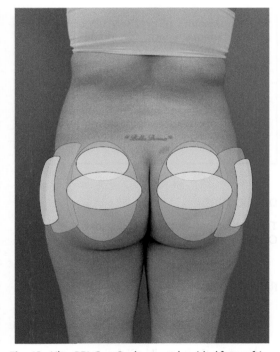

Fig. 13. UltraBBL Case 2: ultrasound-guided fat grafting plan. Gluteal fat grafting was planned to the deep subcutaneous spaces (green) to increase projection and add volume. Fat grafting to the superficial subcutaneous spaces (yellow) would supplement the deep volume and correct superficial irregularities. (*From* Pazmiño, P. (2020). ultraBBL: Brazilian Butt Lift Using Real-Time Intraoperative Ultrasound Guidance. In: Garcia Jr., O. (eds) Ultrasound-Assisted Liposuction. Springer, Cham. https://doi.org/10.1007/978-3-030-26875-6_10.)

RESULT

The patient received gluteal fat grafting under real-time intraoperative ultrasound visualization. The patient received fat separation without suction and fat extraction under suction of the abdomen, waist, flanks, lower back, and sacral areas. Care was taken to empty the waist and flanks and the supra-sacral triangle concavity. She then received 1000 cc of fat graft per side. A total of 700 cc of fat graft was placed in the deep subcutaneous space (above the deep gluteal fascia and below the superficial gluteal fascia) for the creation of gluteal volume, central dome projection, and supra-gluteal contour. Release of adhesions throughout the deep and superficial gluteal spaces at the outer hips was performed, taking care to leave the superficial gluteal fascia intact. She then received 300 cc of fat graft to the superficial subcutaneous space (above the superficial gluteal fascia and below the skin) at the outer hips, bilaterally. Further adhesion separation was performed after fat grafting to ensure even distribution of the fat graft in both spaces. The patient is shown with a 9-month result and is satisfied with the result (**Fig. 14**).

SUMMARY

Gluteal fat grafting is a powerful body contouring technique that can create impressive results not obtainable with implants or liposuction alone. This procedure is very technique dependent and because of the too frequent fatal complications, it

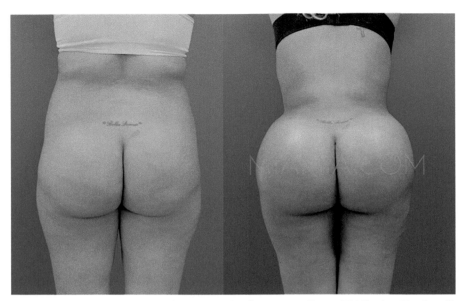

Fig. 14. UltraBBL Case 2. Postoperative result at 9 months. (*From* Pazmiño, P. (2020). ultraBBL: Brazilian Butt Lift Using Real-Time Intraoperative Ultrasound Guidance. In: Garcia Jr., O. (eds) Ultrasound-Assisted Liposuction. Springer, Cham. https://doi.org/10.1007/978-3-030-26875-6_10.)

has been recommended that surgeons avoid intramuscular injection and only fat graft in the subcutaneous space above the deep gluteal fascia. The subcutaneous space, however, is a thin curving dome that ranges in thickness from 1 cm at the outer hips to 3 to 4 cm at the central gluteal dome. This creates a difficult target for gluteal surgeons who do not use intraoperative imaging. Real-time intraoperative ultrasound-guided fat grafting allows the surgeon to consistently avoid an intramuscular injection and manipulate the subcutaneous spaces above and below the superficial gluteal fascia to precisely control fat graft volume and distribution, create projection, and correct superficial irregularities. The surgeon can also create ultrasound video of the entire procedure to document that they remained above the deep gluteal fascia at all times and analyze how their fat graft placement affected their ultimate clinical results. None of this is possible without ultrasound. Real-time intraoperative ultrasound is now an affordable tool that can work with any fat grafting system that can not only make a Brazilian butt lift more accurate and powerful, but safer, as well.

CLINICS CARE POINTS

- Use ultrasound to identify subcutaneous target areas for gluteal fat grafting
- Use ultrasound to always confirm the tip of the cannula is above the deep gluteal fascia before injecting fat graft

- Use ultrasound to precisely target the deep subcutaneous space for dome projection and height
- Use ultrasound to precisely target the superficial subcutaneous space for correction of superficial contour irregularities
- Use ultrasound to measure the height of the subcutaneous spaces before and after injection to document expansion and gluteal projection

DISCLOSURE

The author has nothing to disclose. Consultant: Clarius Mobile Health.

REFERENCES

1. Roberts TL, Toledo LS, Badin AZ. Augmentation of the buttocks by micro fat grafting. Aesthet Surg J 2001;21(4):311–9.
2. Mendieta C, Stuzin JM. Gluteal augmentation and enhancement of the female silhouette: analysis and technique. Plast Reconstr Surg 2018;141(2):306–11.
3. Mofid MM, Teitelbaum S, Suissa D, et al. Report on mortality from gluteal fat grafting: recommendations from the ASERF Task Force. Aesthet Surg J 2017; 37(7):796–806.
4. Wall S, Vecchio D Del. Commentary on: report on mortality from gluteal fat grafting: recommendations

from the ASERF Task Force. Aesthet Surg J 2017; 37(7):807–10.

5. Saylan Z. Liposhifting instead of lipofilling: treatment of postlipoplasty irregularities. Aesthet Surg J 2001; 21(2):137–41.

6. Abboud MH, Dibo SA, Abboud NM. Power-assisted gluteal augmentation: a new technique for sculpting, harvesting, and transferring fat. Aesthet Surg J 2015;35(8):987–94.

7. Wall SH, Lee MR. Separation, aspiration, and fat equalization: SAFE liposuction concepts for comprehensive body contouring. Plast Reconstr Surg 2016; 138(6):1192–201.

8. Condé-Green A, Kotamarti V, Nini KT, et al. Fat grafting for gluteal augmentation: a systematic review of the literature and meta-analysis. Plast Reconstr Surg 2016;138(3):437e–46e.

9. Rapkiewicz AV, Kenerson K, Hutchins KD, et al. Fatal complications of aesthetic techniques: the gluteal region. J Forensic Sci 2018;63(5):1406–12.

10. Villanueva NL, Del Vecchio DA, Afrooz PN, et al. Staying safe during gluteal fat transplantation. Plast Reconstr Surg 2018;141(1):79–86.

11. Villanueva NL, Del Vecchio DA, Afrooz PN, et al. Reply: staying safe during gluteal fat transplantation. Plast Reconstr Surg 2018;142(4):594E–5E.

12. Cárdenas-Camarena L, Bayter JE, Aguirre-Serrano H, et al. Deaths caused by gluteal lipoinjection: what are we doing wrong? Plast Reconstr Surg 2015;136(1):58–66.

13. Turin SY, Fracol M, Keller E, et al. Gluteal vein anatomy: location, caliber, impact of patient positioning, and implications for fat grafting. Aesthet Surg J 2020;40(6):642–9.

14. Pazmiño P, Garcia O. Brazilian butt lift–associated mortality: the South Florida experience. Aesthet Surg J 2022. https://doi.org/10.1093/ASJ/SJAC224.

15. Mills D, Rubin P, Saltz R. 2018.07 Urgent Warning to Surgeons Performing Fat Grafting to the Buttocks Brazilian Butt Lift or "BBL". Published July 18, 2018. Available at: https://www.plasticsurgery.org/documents/Patient-Safety/BBL/Gluteal-Fat-Grafting-Safety-Advisory_Jul18.pdf. Accessed June 26, 2023.

16. Mills D, Rubin P, Saltz R. 2018.01 Multisociety Gluteal Fat Grafting Task Force Issues Safety Advisory Urging Practitioners to Reevaluate Technique. Published online January 31, 2018. Available at: https://www.plasticsurgery.org/documents/Patient-Safety/BBL/Gluteal-Fat-Grafting-Safety-Advisory_Jan18.pdf. Accessed June 26, 2023.

17. Rios L, Gupta V. Improvement in Brazilian butt lift (BBL) safety with the current recommendations from ASERF, ASAPS, and ISAPS. Aesthet Surg J 2020;40(8):864–70.

18. Cansancao AL, Condé-Green A, Vidigal RA, et al. Real-time ultrasound-assisted gluteal fat grafting. Plast Reconstr Surg 2018;142(2):372–6.

19. Pazmiño P, Del Vecchio D. Static injection, migration, and equalization (sime): a new paradigm for safe ultrasound-guided Brazilian butt lift: safer, faster, better. Aesthet Surg J 2023. https://doi.org/10.1093/ASJ/SJAD142.

20. Lucas VS, Burk RS, Creehan S, et al. Utility of high-frequency ultrasound: moving beyond the surface to detect changes in skin integrity. Plast Surg Nurs 2014;34(1):34.

21. Shermak M. Body Contouring. Published 2011. Available at: https://books.google.com/books?id=LmUWgPpOBAwC&printsec=frontcover&source=gbs_ge_summary_r&cad=0#v=onepage&q&f=false. Accessed June 26, 2023

22. Stecco C, Hammer W, Vleeming A, et al. Subcutaneous tissue and superficial fascia. Functional Atlas of the Human Fascial System 2015;1:21–49.

23. Del Vecchio DA, Villanueva NL, Mohan R, et al. Clinical implications of gluteal fat graft migration: a dynamic anatomical study. Plast Reconstr Surg 2018; 142(5):1180–92.

24. Frojo G, Halani SH, Pessa JE, et al. Deep subcutaneous gluteal fat compartments: anatomy and clinical implications. Aesthet Surg J 2023;43(1): 76–83.

25. Del Vecchio D, Wall S. Expansion vibration lipofilling: a new technique in large-volume fat transplantation. Plast Reconstr Surg 2018;141(5):639e–49e.

26. Del Vecchio D, Wall S, Stein MJ, et al. Simultaneous separation and tumescence: a new paradigm for liposuction donor site preparation. Aesthet Surg J 2022;42(12):1427–32.

27. Urgent warning to surgeons performing fat grafting to the buttocks (Brazilian Butt Lift or "BBL").

Static Injection, Migration, and Equalization
A New Paradigm for Safe Ultrasound-Guided BBL: Safer, Faster, Better

Pat Pazmiño, MD[a],*, Daniel Del Vecchio, MD, MBA[b]

KEYWORDS

- SIME • Static injection • Migration and equalization • Brazilian butt lift • BBL • Gluteal fat grafting
- Buttock augmentation • Buttock enlargement

KEY POINTS

- Ultrasound allows surgeons to specifically target the superficial or deep subcutaneous space for fat grafting.
- The privileged anatomy of the deep subcutaneous space allows for lateral migration of fat graft even with a static cannula.
- After static injection, fat graft can be distributed, as needed via equalization with a moving cannula.
- Static injection, migration, and equalization can precisely place fat graft in the deep and the superficial subcutaneous spaces.

INTRODUCTION

During the past 5 years, gluteal fat grafting, commonly referred to as a Brazilian butt lift, or "BBL" has been one of the most popular and controversial procedures in esthetic surgery.[1,2] Although it can produce dramatic results, the consequences are sometimes fatal if not done correctly.

Multiple plastic surgery societies (ASAPS, ASPS, ISAPS, ISPRES, and IFATS) published guidelines that emphasized that fat graft must only be injected above the muscle in the subcutaneous layer.[3]

These guidelines and laws appropriately describe *where* the fat graft should be placed but

they do not show surgeons *how* to accurately and consistently inject fat graft in the subcutaneous space. This lack of total certainty as to the safe and correct placement of fat graft is the final obstacle in making the BBL safe, efficient, accurate, consistent, and teachable.

Materials and Methods

The authors performed more than 4200 BBLs using ultrasound-assisted gluteal fat grafting from May 2013 to December 2022. Each BBL with ultrasound-assisted gluteal fat grafting was performed by a single surgeon. Patients' age ranged from 18 to 69 years with an average age of 34.2 years and an average body mass index of

This article is an update of a previously published article by the same authors in *Aesthetic Surgery Journal*.
[a] Division of Plastic Surgery, University of Miami, 848 Brickell Avenue, Suite 820, Miami, FL 33131, USA;
[b] Department of Plastic Surgery, Massachusetts General Hospital, 38 Newbury Street, Suite 502, Boston, MA 02116, USA
* Corresponding author.
E-mail address: cps@miamia.com

plasticsurgery.theclinics.com

31.3. Eight different ultrasound systems were used including the CE Ultrasound (Beijing, China), Interson SeeMore (Pleasanton, CA), Philips Lumify L12 to 4 (Andover, MA), Butterfly iQ (Burlington, MA), PS-Imaging (Grand Rapids, MI), Clarius L7 and L15 (Vancouver, BC), and GE Vscan (Chicago, IL).

Essential Gluteal Soft Tissue Anatomy—Two Fasciae and Two Fat Layers

Radiology and surgical anatomy literature have long described 2 distinct subcutaneous fasciae throughout the human body: a thinner, elastic, areolar fascia called the superficial fascia (eg, Scarpa fascia in the anterior abdomen) that divides the subcutaneous zone into 2 distinct spaces and a thicker, inelastic fascia called the deep fascia (eg, rectus fascia in the anterior abdomen) that invests the surface of the muscles. These 2 fasciae are morphologically, histologically, and functionally distinct.[4-8]

Both of these subcutaneous fascial layers also exist throughout the gluteal region (**Fig. 1**). The superficial gluteal fascia (SGF), which lies below the dermis and above the muscles, is a part of the superficial fascial system and is analogous to Scarpa fascia throughout the anterior abdomen. There is also a deep gluteal fascia (DGF), which is the muscular fascia that invests the external surface of the gluteus maximus muscle.[9]

The DGF is a single thick layer of fascia attached to the underlying gluteus maximus, whereas the SGF is impregnated with fat globules and has the appearance of bubble wrap on gross dissection. The SGF is clinically relevant because it divides the subcutaneous zone into 2 distinct subcutaneous spaces: the superficial subcutaneous space (between the dermis and the SGF) and the deep subcutaneous space (between the SGF and the DGF) (**Fig. 2**).[6] The superficial subcutaneous space is more organized and demonstrates segmental palisades of dermo-fascial attachments, whereas fat in the deep subcutaneous space demonstrates a less-dense fibroseptal network. This nuanced anatomic difference is critical and serves as the basis for static injection, migration, and equalization (SIME).

Ultrasound allows the surgeon to visually appreciate these fascial layers and to accurately target these 2 distinct subcutaneous spaces in the operating room (**Fig. 3**).

The DGF is clinically relevant because dynamic cadaver studies have demonstrated that if fat graft is injected above an intact DGF or a DGF with small defects (defects smaller than 1 cm), the DGF acts like a "stout wall," preventing subcutaneous fat graft from migrating into or under the gluteus maximus muscle.[10] This cadaver study demonstrated that fat graft only migrated through the DGF when 1 cm or larger sections were surgically excised from the DGF. Preventing fat graft from migrating into the gluteal muscles will also stop fat graft from reaching the gluteal veins, thus preventing a fatal pulmonary fat embolism. Surgeons should take comfort from these findings because small perforations in the DGF caused by an inadvertent cannula are not large enough to allow subcutaneous fat graft to migrate into the gluteal muscles. Surgeons who can confirm subcutaneous fat graft placement can perform this procedure safely. All autopsies of BBL patients who perished from pulmonary fat emboli (PFE) have the common finding of fat graft within the gluteal muscles, emphasizing the importance of avoiding intramuscular fat graft placement.[11] These research and autopsy findings were the foundation of the 2018 Joint Society Task Force guidelines that recommended surgeons only inject fat graft subcutaneously, above the DGF.[3,12]

It is important to remember that the entire subcutaneous zone (from the dermis to the DGF) varies from patient to patient and can range in thickness from 1 cm at the lateral hip to 3 cm or greater at the gluteal dome.[13,14] Surgeons, therefore, must graft within a thin curved dome of varying thickness. The technical challenge of consistently remaining in this thin, irregular, variable space may account for the inadvertent deep intramuscular injections by well-intentioned surgeons performing fat grafting without ultrasound visualization.

Description of the SIME Technique—Static Injection, Migration, and Equalization

Previous descriptions of ultrasound-guided fat grafting used 2 operators—a first operator who would perform the fat injection with a cannula in constant motion and a second operator who would follow the moving injection cannula in tandem with an ultrasound probe.[15]

The subtle nuance of a *static approach* to both the injecting cannula and the ultrasound probe was first conceived and described by the author (Pazmiño) and is outlined below. The ultrasound probe is placed on the skin over the first site that will receive fat graft, typically the central buttock dome. The injection cannula is inserted through a skin incision and advanced to the first injection site just underneath the ultrasound probe and remains stationary. Ultrasound confirms the cannula's position above the DGF and below the SGF within the deep subcutaneous space (**Fig. 4**A). The cannula remains stationary and fat

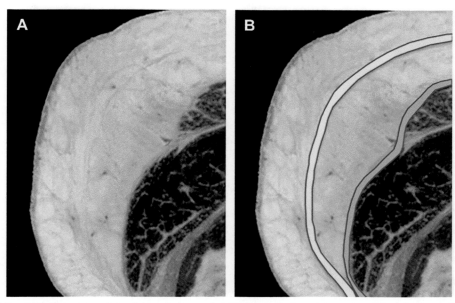

Fig. 1. (*A*) Transverse cross section of female buttocks. (*B*) Transverse cross section of female buttocks. The SGF (yellow) is below the dermis and above the DGF and divides the subcutaneous region into 2 distinct spaces. The DGF (green) lies on the external surface of the gluteus maximus muscle. (*From* Pazmiño, P. (2020). ultraBBL: Brazilian Butt Lift Using Real-Time Intraoperative Ultrasound Guidance. In: Garcia Jr., O. (eds) Ultrasound-Assisted Liposuction. Springer, Cham. https://doi.org/10.1007/978-3-030-26875-6_10.)

graft is injected (*Static injection*). By confirming that the fat graft is only injected in the deep subcutaneous space, we can exploit the principle of subcutaneous migration (SUM) and visualize the fat graft filling this contained space until an esthetic endpoint is achieved (**Fig.** 4B) (*Migration*).[12] The ultrasound probe is then placed on the skin over the next injection site. The cannula is then advanced under the ultrasound probe remaining in the deep subcutaneous space. Once the ultrasound confirms the new cannula position above the DGF, fat graft is then injected into this second site (**Fig.** 4C). The technique is repeated along multiple points around the gluteal dome until esthetic lipofilling has been achieved. After all the desired fat graft volume has been placed in the deep subcutaneous space, *and with no further fat injection*, the surgeon can move the cannula in a dynamic fashion as necessary to distribute the fat graft and smooth irregularities (**Fig.** 4D), using the equalization concept (*Equalization*) first described by Wall in his classic SAFE Lipo communication.[16] It should be noted that gluteal fat grafting via SIME is not limited to the deep subcutaneous space. Although the majority of fat graft volume will be placed in the deep subcutaneous space, ultrasound allows the surgeon to selectively enter the narrow superficial subcutaneous

space and inject fat graft when correction of superficial contour irregularities is necessary or to produce additional projection in selected sites.

It is the unique and privileged anatomy of the deep subcutaneous space—with a relative paucity of connective tissue—that allows for the migration of fat using static injection, without the creation of a bolus deposition. In the SIME surgical plan, fat is first inserted under the central dome, then to multiple sites laterally until the "C point" described by Mendieta[17,18] is reached, and ultimately at the lower outer quadrant of the gluteal region, inferolateral to the infragluteal crease. After all fat graft has been injected, the surgeon can use a moving cannula to disperse fat graft and smooth any contour irregularities (*Equalization*) (**Figs.** 5–7). It is important to note that fat graft is only injected under ultrasound visualization and never when the cannula is in motion.

Results

Complications included 5 infections (0.12%), 180 seromas (4.3%), 30 unfavorable (hypertrophic) scars (0.7%), 18 fat necrosis cases (0.4%), 27 lipid cysts (0.7%), 25 cases of excess fat absorption (0.6%), 72 cases of asymmetry (1.7%), and 90 contour irregularities (2.2%). Eighty-one patients

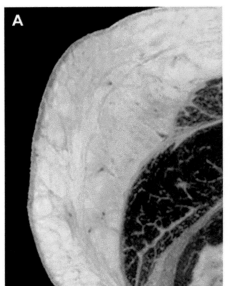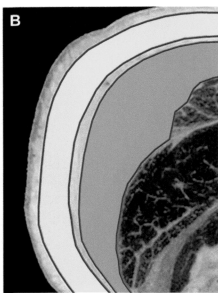

Fig. 2. (*A*) Transverse cross section of female buttocks. (*B*) Transverse cross section of female buttocks. The SGF divides the subcutaneous zone into 2 spaces. The *superficial* subcutaneous space (yellow) is below the dermis and above the SGF. The *deep* subcutaneous space (green) is below the SGF and above the DGF. Ultrasound allows the surgeon to accurately enter each space and manipulate it while always remaining above the DGF. Note the differences in connective tissue density and organization between the superficial subcutaneous space and the deep subcutaneous space. Clinically, the preferred fat grafting space is the *deep* subcutaneous space, due to its deeper position and its less dense fibroseptal network that permits the smooth subcutaneous migration of grafted fat. (*From* Pazmiño, P. (2020). ultraBBL: Brazilian Butt Lift Using Real-Time Intraoperative Ultrasound Guidance. In: Garcia Jr., O. (eds) Ultrasound-Assisted Liposuction. Springer, Cham. https://doi.org/10.1007/978-3-030-26875-6_10.)

(1.95%) required revision surgery to correct irregularities from asymmetric fat absorption and 675 patients (16.3%) elected to receive a secondary BBL to further augment gluteal volume and projection. There were no instances of burns or skin changes from the ultrasound probe, no deep venous thrombi, no thromboembolic pulmonary emboli, no fat pulmonary emboli, and no critical care admissions, or deaths.

On occasion, both surgeons noted that after the initial insertion of the cannula, the ultrasound probe revealed that the cannula tip was *under the DGF* and within the muscle body of the gluteus maximus. In these instances, the ultrasound alerted the surgeon to recognize this incorrect cannula position, withdraw the cannula, place it correctly above the DGF before any fat graft was deployed. This is a critical safety feature of using real-time intraoperative ultrasound for gluteal fat grafting.

DISCUSSION

During the last 10 years, our understanding of the principles of gluteal fat grafting and our surgical techniques has dramatically evolved. In 2015, Cárdenas-Camarena and colleagues collected the experience of plastic surgeons in Mexico and Colombia during the past 10 and 15 years, respectively, and identified 13 PFE deaths in Mexico and 9 PFE deaths in Colombia after gluteal fat grafting. They reviewed the autopsy findings and found that the deaths were associated with intramuscular fat grafting and recommended surgeons avoid fat graft injections into the deep muscle planes.[19] Mofid and colleagues performed an online surgeon survey and raised the alarm that PFE deaths were happening in the United States as well with a seemingly high number coming from Florida.[20] The state of Florida represents 6.5% of the US population[21] but represents more than 28% of the US deaths from BBL. The mortality rate in Florida is 4.3 times what would be expected on a pro rata population basis.

Two dynamic cadaver studies on deep intramuscular migration (DIM) and SUM, referred to as the "DIM SUM" articles, have demonstrated that fat graft injected under the DGF readily migrated throughout and under the gluteus maximus muscle.[10,12] It was also noted that if the

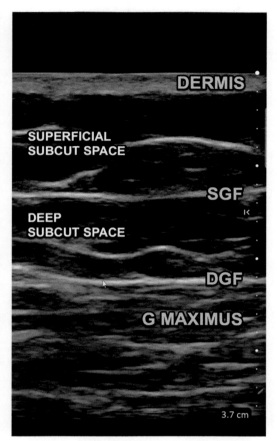

Fig. 3. Ultrasound image of key gluteal anatomic landmarks. The dermis is seen at the top of the image abutting the surface of the ultrasound probe. The striated muscle of the gluteus maximus is at the bottom of the image. The DGF (*white arrow*) is the thick and uniform fascia layer overlying the gluteus maximus muscle. The SGF has the appearance of bubble wrap and is impregnated with fat globules. The SGF divides the subcutaneous zone into the superficial subcutaneous space and the deep subcutaneous space. (*From* Pazmiño P, Del Vecchio D. Static Injection, Migration, and Equalization (SIME): A New Paradigm for Safe Ultrasound-Guided Brazilian Butt Lift: Safer, Faster, Better [published online ahead of print, 2023 May 9]. Aesthet Surg J. 2023;sjad142.)

DGF did not have defects larger than 1 cm, the DGF could act as a "stout wall" to prevent subcutaneous fat graft from extending into the gluteus maximus muscle.[12] These studies highlighted that subcutaneous gluteal fat grafting could be performed safely, as small openings in the DGF caused by a passing cannula were not large enough to allow fat migration below the DGF. These cadaver studies and supporting autopsy findings were the basis of recommending a "subcutaneous only" BBL technique.[22–24]

All of these studies emphasize limiting fat graft to the subcutaneous space; however, the missing link remains—"how does a surgeon ensure that they are subcutaneous and above the DGF at all times?" Real-time intraoperative ultrasound fills this "missing link" by allowing surgeons to confirm their subcutaneous fat graft placement in every case.

Previous descriptions of ultrasound-guided fat grafting recommended a 2-operator approach to visualize continuous cannula movement during fat graft injection.[15] Cannula motion made continuous ultrasound tracking time consuming and difficult. Having 2 different brains trying to work in tandem, one with a cannula and the other with an ultrasound probe, is extremely difficult. As one errant pass of the cannula under the DGF could incite a pulmonary fat embolism, failure to visualize a moving cannula even for a single stroke could leave uncertainty that all of the fat graft had been placed in the correct space.

With the SIME technique, once the correct subcutaneous position of the cannula tip above the DGF has been confirmed, fat graft is injected in a *static manner*. The superficial and DGF remain intact and create a compartment that allows for the dynamic migration of fat through the deep subcutaneous space. Ultrasound allows the surgeon to witness the doubling or tripling in height of this deep subcutaneous space because it fills with fat graft (**Figs. 8** and **9**):

After the deep subcutaneous space has been adequately filled at the first injection site, the surgeon places the ultrasound probe over the next injection site. The surgeon advances the cannula under the ultrasound probe and once the correct position of the cannula above the DGF is confirmed, fat graft is statically injected at the second site. To be clear, there is no cannula motion during fat injection. After the fat graft has been deposited within the deep subcutaneous space at all desired locations, the surgeon can move the cannula to distribute or equalize the fat graft to address any irregularities between the recipient sites, as needed.

When comparing the insertion rates using SIME versus classic nonultrasonic fat grafting, the volume-adjusted insertion rates using SIME were higher and were statistically significant, suggesting SIME is not only a safer technique but is also more time-efficient. Shorter insertion times may stem from the fact that static insertion does not require the operator to move the cannula throughout the recipient site as much, as targeted grafting may be occurring in what may be discrete gluteal fat compartments. Further studies using dynamic cadaver models have been completed and

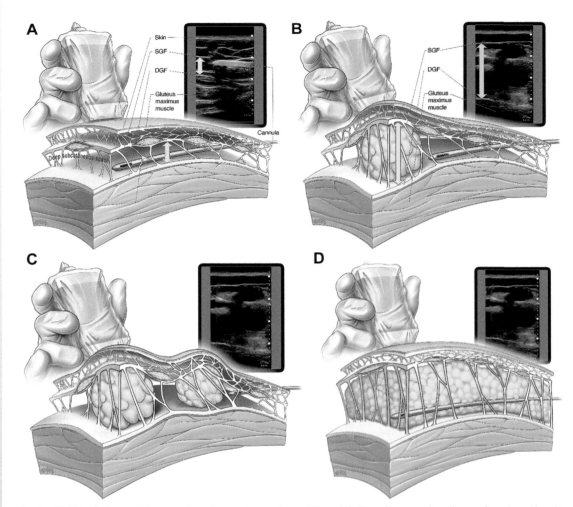

Fig. 4. SIME technique: Ultrasound probe and cannula position. (*A*) The ultrasound probe is placed on the skin over the first site of fat graft injection, typically at the center of the gluteal dome (see **Fig. 5**A). The injection cannula is inserted through the skin and advanced toward the ultrasound probe. The surgeon uses the ultrasound to visualize all subcutaneous structures and confirm the position of the cannula in the deep subcutaneous space, below the SGF and above the DGF. The height of the unexpanded deep subcutaneous space is noted (small yellow double *arrow*). (*B*) Once the cannula position has been confirmed to be above the DGF, the cannula remains stationary and fat graft is injected (Static injection). Fat graft migrates easily through the deep subcutaneous space (Migration). During the injection, the surgeon assesses the external gluteal contour and stops the static injection when sufficient gluteal projection has been achieved. The ultrasound will confirm a doubling or tripling of the height of the deep subcutaneous space (large yellow double *arrow*). (*C*) Once the desired projection and esthetic endpoint of the first site has been achieved, the ultrasound probe is moved to the next injection site. The cannula is again advanced to the probe. Once the position of the cannula has been confirmed to be above the DGF, the cannula remains stationary and fat graft is injected at the second site (see **Fig. 5**B). (*D*) After all sites have been injected, the surgeon can use the cannula in a dynamic fashion to equalize the fat graft between the areas of injected fat to correct irregularities (Equalization). Fat graft is only injected under ultrasound visualization and never when the cannula is in motion. (*From* Pazmiño P, Del Vecchio D. Static Injection, Migration, and Equalization (SIME): A New Paradigm for Safe Ultrasound-Guided Brazilian Butt Lift: Safer, Faster, Better [published online ahead of print, 2023 May 9]. Aesthet Surg J. 2023;sjad142.)

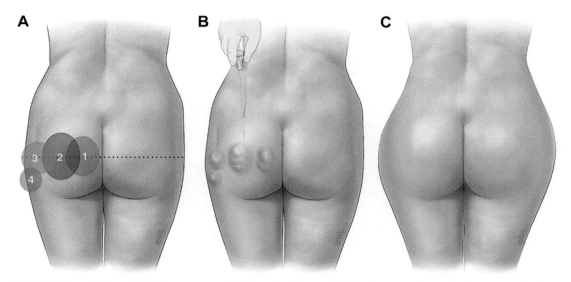

Fig. 5. SIME technique: Injection strategy. (*A*) Sites for fat graft injection are determined preoperatively to achieve gluteal dome projection and lateral hip fullness. Fat graft is first placed with a static cannula under ultrasound visualization in the deep subcutaneous space in the central dome compartment (1 and 2). The cannula is then moved to a new position laterally along the transverse line from the midportion of the natal cleft to the desired point of maximum projection at the lateral hip. Fat graft is injected at these sites with a static cannula under ultrasound visualization (3). Fat graft can be injected in the inferolateral hip as needed (4). Ultrasound is used to confirm that a static cannula is above the DGF during all stationary fat grafting (Static injection). Fat graft migrates smoothly through the deep subcutaneous space (Migration). (*B*) After all sites have been injected, it is common for the external surface to appear bumpy or irregular. (*C*) A moving cannula can be used to distribute injected fat graft between these sites and create a smooth final contour (Equalization). (*From* Pazmiño P, Del Vecchio D. Static Injection, Migration, and Equalization (SIME): A New Paradigm for Safe Ultrasound-Guided Brazilian Butt Lift: Safer, Faster, Better [published online ahead of print, 2023 May 9]. Aesthet Surg J. 2023;sjad142.)

delineate the nature, size, and location of these apparent deep subcutaneous compartments.[25] Guidelines released earlier this year emphasized the role of surgeon awareness in the subcutaneous space and the use of ultrasound to confirm proper cannula tip location and placement of fat graft in all BBL cases.[23]

Targeted Compartmental Grafting and "Fascia Preservation"

Safe and effective fat transplantation requires accurate placement of the cannula and grafted fat in the deep subcutaneous space, keeping the DGF and the SGF intact. Such precise placement is only possible using ultrasound visualization. Targeting the deep subcutaneous space and using "fascia preservation" allows the surgeon to take advantage of the dynamic migration characteristics of this unique space and allows for greater projection with lower overall volumes than had previously been accomplished when fat was not preferentially solely in the deep

subcutaneous layer. By avoiding fat placement in the superficial subcutaneous fat layer, one also avoids a flattened "discoid" appearance of the dome and a *peau d'orange* effect on the skin. Such esthetic disharmonies are a manifestation of fat being above the SGF in superficial subcutaneous space with its dense fibroseptal network that results in sluggish and irregular horizontal migration of fat.

This nuanced expansion vibration lipofilling (EVL) derivative, *Static Injection, Migration, and Equalization*, is coined "SIME" and can only be performed under ultrasound guidance. Ultrasound not only allows for the confirmation of safe subcutaneous fat graft placement but also allows the surgeon to maintain the integrity of both gluteal fasciae so that these structures can guide the subcutaneous migration of the fat graft. Without ultrasound, fat graft could be inadvertently placed under the DGF and into the muscle, exposing the patient to the risk of a pulmonary fat embolism.[11,26] Without ultrasound, the SGF could be disrupted. If the SGF remains intact, it

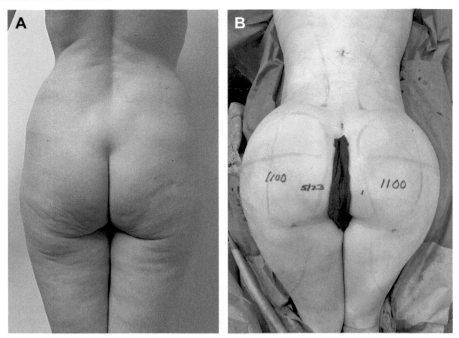

Fig. 6. (*A*) Preoperative view: A 36-year-old woman interested in gluteal augmentation and contouring. (*B*) Post-operative "On Table" view: BBL using SIME technique (DDV). Note the relatively low volumes required to achieve satisfactory postero-lateral projection and smoothness of contours. DDV, Daniel Del Vecchio. (*From* Pazmiño P, Del Vecchio D. Static Injection, Migration, and Equalization (SIME): A New Paradigm for Safe Ultrasound-Guided Brazilian Butt Lift: Safer, Faster, Better [published online ahead of print, 2023 May 9]. Aesthet Surg J. 2023;sjad142.)

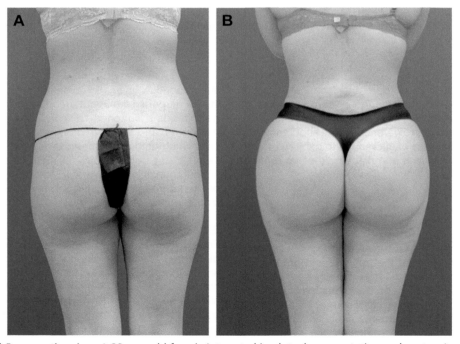

Fig. 7. (*A*) Preoperative view: A 28-year-old female interested in gluteal augmentation and contouring. (*B*) Post-operative 12-month view: SIME BBL after 900 cc of fat injected per buttock (PP). Note the dramatic change in the hip-to-waist ratio and the relatively low volumes required to achieve satisfactory postero-lateral projection and smoothness of contours. (*From* Pazmiño P, Del Vecchio D. Static Injection, Migration, and Equalization (SIME): A New Paradigm for Safe Ultrasound-Guided Brazilian Butt Lift: Safer, Faster, Better [published online ahead of print, 2023 May 9]. Aesthet Surg J. 2023;sjad142.)

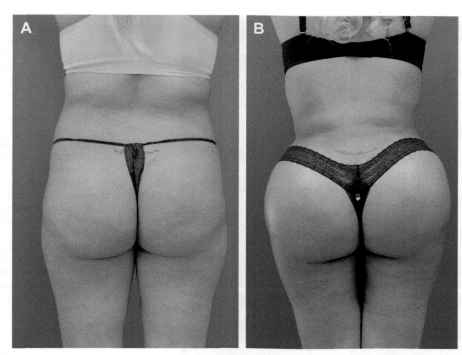

Fig. 8. (*A*) Preoperative view: A 31-year-old woman interested in gluteal augmentation and contouring. Image used with permission from: Pazmiño P. (*B*) Postoperative 12-month view: SIME BBL after 1100 cc of fat was injected per buttock (PP). Note the firmness and fullness of the buttocks when fat is placed as deep as possible in the deep subcutaneous space. (*From* Pazmiño P, Del Vecchio D. Static Injection, Migration, and Equalization (SIME): A New Paradigm for Safe Ultrasound-Guided Brazilian Butt Lift: Safer, Faster, Better [published online ahead of print, 2023 May 9]. Aesthet Surg J. 2023;sjad142.)

can retain the fat graft that is specifically injected below it, like the casing of a sausage. Fat graft injected into this deep subcutaneous space can act similar to a subfascial implant, creating excellent volumetric augmentation and central dome projection. Fat graft injected into the superficial subcutaneous space (below the dermis and above the SGF) in the central gluteus can flatten the gluteal dome and can also potentially lead to "blow out" fat fractures, skin changes, and surface irregularities. Ultrasound guidance can allow the surgeon to selectively target the superficial space to correct minor superficial contour deformities and depressions but superficial subcutaneous space grafting is not relied on for large volume or large contour changes, per se.

Benefits of the SIME technique include accurate fat graft placement, more efficient grafting with shorter injection times, smaller volumes of fat required to achieve an overall esthetic result, and 100% certainty that the fat graft has only been placed in the subcutaneous space and above the DGF. Video documentation of the procedure and of the operating surgeon with a self-facing camera also serves to memorialize the procedure's safe execution and visual identification of the operating surgeon. Intraoperative ultrasound images and video can be recorded and may also be saved as part of the patient's medical record.

Limitations of SIME and ultrasound-guided fat grafting include the one-time purchase of the ultrasound equipment (less than US$4000) and the learning curve of 3 to 5 cases as surgeons familiarize themselves with the new equipment and practice the coordination of the ultrasound probe and the fat grafting cannula.

The SIME technique represents a further evolution of Wall's SAFE Lipo principles[16] and is a fusion of 3 body-contouring benchmarks: SAFE Lipo, EVL, and ultrasound-guided BBL. The SIME technique of ultrasound-guided BBL ensures the safe placement of fat graft above the muscle, allows for more efficient fat grafting with less cannula motion, and better control in gluteal shaping.

In short, it is "safer, faster, and better."

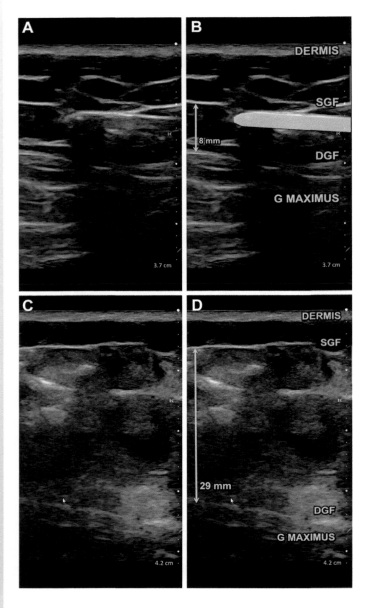

Fig. 9. SIME case (*A*) Preinjection original sonogram: The cannula is noted within the deep subcutaneous space directly beneath the SGF. The deep subcutaneous space has a preinjection height of 8 mm. Note the sonographic shadow artifact obscuring the view of the deeper structures beneath the cannula. (*B*) Preinjection annotated sonogram. (*C*) Postinjection original: Injected fat graft has now filled the deep subcutaneous space and displaced the DGF downward and the SGF upward. Both fasciae remain intact and the height of the deep subcutaneous space has now increased by a factor of 3.6. (*D*) Postinjection annotated sonogram. (*From* Pazmiño P, Del Vecchio D. Static Injection, Migration, and Equalization (SIME): A New Paradigm for Safe Ultrasound-Guided Brazilian Butt Lift: Safer, Faster, Better [published online ahead of print, 2023 May 9]. Aesthet Surg J. 2023;sjad142.)

SUMMARY

SIME represents the missing link in performing safe subcutaneous buttock augmentation. Training in real-time intraoperative ultrasound is recommended for residents and practicing surgeons who perform gluteal fat grafting.[23] Through a better understanding of the pathophysiology of pulmonary fat embolism, a better appreciation of the migrational properties of grafted fat, identifying safe and unsafe recipient sites, targeting distinct compartments in the deep subcutaneous space, and through technical refinements in ultrasound-guided fat transplantation, surgeons now have the necessary tools to perform gluteal fat grafting in a safe, efficient, and accurate manner. This will lead to a decreased overall mortality rate for this procedure, approaching that of liposuction, and will allow surgeons to offer a safer procedure for their patients.

CLINICS CARE POINTS

- Once ultrasound has confirmed the cannula tip position above the DGF, injecting fat graft without moving the cannula will ensure consistent subcutaneous fat grafting (Static injection)
- Take advantage of the less dense tissue in the deep subcutaneous spaces to allow the fat graft to migrate laterally (Migration)
- After static fat graft injection, use a moving cannula to disperse fat graft, correct contour irregularities, as needed
- Use SIME to create excellent gluteal projection with fat graft in the deep subcutaneous space
- Use SIME to correct superficial contour irregularities with fat graft in the superficial subcutaneous space

DISCLOSURE

Consultant: Clarius Mobile Health.

REFERENCES

1. The Aesthetic Society. Aesthetic plastic surgery national databank 2021. Aesthet Surg J 2022;42(Supp 1):1–18.
2. Ghavami A, Villanueva NL. Gluteal augmentation and contouring with autologous fat transfer: Part I. Clin Plast Surg 2018;45(2):249–59. https://doi.org/10.1016/j.cps.2017.12.009.
3. Mills D, Rubin P, Saltz R. Fat grafting to the buttocks. American Society of Plastic Surgeons. ASPS; 2018. Available at: https://www.plasticsurgery.org/for-medical-professionals/advocacy/key-issues/fat-grafting-to-the-buttocks. Accessed July 24, 2022.
4. Gatt A, Agarwal S, Zito P. Anatomy, fascia layers. StatPearls; 2021. Available at: https://pubmed.ncbi.nlm.nih.gov/30252294/. Accessed July 24, 2022.
5. O'Leary C. Fasciae of the hip and thigh: Anatomy | Kenhub. KenHub. Available at: https://www.kenhub.com/en/library/anatomy/fasciae-of-the-hip-and-thigh. Accessed July 24, 2022.
6. Stecco C, Porzionato A, Lancerotto L, et al. Histological study of the deep fasciae of the limbs. J Bodyw Mov Ther 2008;12(3):225–30. https://doi.org/10.1016/J.JBMT.2008.04.041.
7. Lee S, Joo K bin, Song SY. Accurate definition of superficial and deep fascia. Radiology 2011;261(3):994. https://doi.org/10.1148/RADIOL.11111116.
8. Benjamin M. The fascia of the limbs and back–a review. J Anat 2009;214(1):1–18. https://doi.org/10.1111/J.1469-7580.2008.01011.X.
9. Pazmiño P. ultraBBL: Brazilian Butt Lift using real-time intraoperative ultrasound guidance. Ultrasound-Assisted Liposuction 2020;147–72. https://doi.org/10.1007/978-3-030-26875-6_10.
10. del Vecchio DA, Villanueva NL, Mohan R, et al. Clinical implications of gluteal fat graft migration: a dynamic anatomical study. Plast Reconstr Surg 2018;142(5):1180–92. https://doi.org/10.1097/PRS.0000000000005020.
11. Pazmiño P, Garcia O. Brazilian Butt lift–associated mortality: the south Florida experience. Aesthet Surg J 2022. https://doi.org/10.1093/ASJ/SJAC224.
12. Wall S, del Vecchio D, Teitelbaum S, et al. Subcutaneous migration: a dynamic anatomical study of gluteal fat grafting. Plast Reconstr Surg 2019;143(5):1343–51. https://doi.org/10.1097/PRS.0000000000005521.
13. Cansancao AL, Condé-Green A, David JA, et al. Subcutaneous-only gluteal fat grafting: a prospective study of the long-term results with ultrasound analysis. Plast Reconstr Surg 2019;143(2):447–51. https://doi.org/10.1097/PRS.0000000000005203.
14. Turin SY, Fracol M, Keller E, et al. Gluteal vein anatomy: location, caliber, impact of patient positioning, and implications for fat grafting. Aesthet Surg J 2020;40(6):642–9. https://doi.org/10.1093/ASJ/SJZ260.
15. Cansancao AL, Condé-Green A, Vidigal RA, et al. Real-time ultrasound-assisted gluteal fat grafting. Plast Reconstr Surg 2018;142(2):372–6. https://doi.org/10.1097/PRS.0000000000004602.
16. Wall SH, Lee MR. Separation, aspiration, and fat equalization: SAFE liposuction concepts for comprehensive body contouring. Plast Reconstr Surg 2016;138(6):1192–201. https://doi.org/10.1097/PRS.0000000000002808.
17. Mendieta C. The Art of Gluteal Sculpting.; 2011. https://www.thieme.in/the-art-of-gluteal-sculpting. Accessed July 24, 2022.
18. Mendieta C, Stuzin JM. Gluteal augmentation and enhancement of the female silhouette: analysis and technique. Plast Reconstr Surg 2018;141(2):306–11. https://doi.org/10.1097/PRS.0000000000004094.
19. Cárdenas-Camarena L, Bayter JE, Aguirre-Serrano H, et al. Deaths caused by gluteal lipoinjection: what are we doing wrong? Plast Reconstr Surg 2015;136(1):58–66. https://doi.org/10.1097/PRS.0000000000001364.
20. Mofid MM, Teitelbaum S, Suissa D, et al. Report on mortality from gluteal fat grafting: recommendations from the ASERF Task Force. Aesthet Surg J 2017;37(7):796. https://doi.org/10.1093/ASJ/SJX004.
21. InfoPlease. U.S. State Populations by Rank. InfoPlease. 2021. Available at: https://www.infoplease.

com/us/states/state-population-by-rank. Accessed July 24, 2022.

22. del Vecchio D. Common sense for the common good: staying subcutaneous during fat transplantation to the gluteal region. Plast Reconstr Surg 2018;142(1):286–8. https://doi.org/10.1097/PRS.0000000000004541.

23. del Vecchio D, Kenkel JM. Practice advisory on gluteal fat grafting. Aesthet Surg J 2022. https://doi.org/10.1093/ASJ/SJAC082.

24. del Vecchio DA, Rohrich RJ. A changing Paradigm: the Brazilian Butt Lift is neither Brazilian nor a lift-why it needs to Be called safe subcutaneous buttock augmentation. Plast Reconstr Surg 2020;145(1):281–3. https://doi.org/10.1097/PRS.0000000000006369.

25. Frojo G, Halani SH, Pessa JE, et al. Deep subcutaneous gluteal fat compartments: anatomy and clinical implications. Aesthet Surg J 2022. https://doi.org/10.1093/ASJ/SJAC230.

26. Ramírez-Montañana A. Commentary on: deep subcutaneous gluteal fat compartments: anatomy and clinical implications. Aesthet Surg J 2022. https://doi.org/10.1093/ASJ/SJAC242.

Gluteal Augmentation in Men

Neil M. Vranis, MD[a],*, Douglas Steinbrech, MD[b]

KEYWORDS

- Male buttock sculpting • Male gluteal augmentation • Body contouring • Gluteal autoaugmentation
- Male gluteal implants

KEY POINTS

- Regardless of technique, avoid lateral buttock expansion in men, which leads to a more rounded, feminine appearance.
- During fat transfer/BodyBanking for the purpose of male gluteal enhancement, the inferior and superior poles in addition to the central region are augmented achieving a vertical, oblong shape.
- An inferiorly based vertical turnover flap can be used for gluteal autoaugmentation in men who present with significant skin laxity after massive weight loss.
- Properly placed subfascial or intramuscular implants can enhance buttock shape, projection, and contours with a reasonable safety profile.
- Combinations of gluteal implants, regional liposuction, fat transfer, and local tissue rearrangement can be performed to optimize the aesthetic result for each patient.

INTRODUCTION

As Male Plastic Surgery becomes increasingly popular and more accepted in modern day society, the demand for male gluteal enhancement procedures parallels this demand. Several techniques have been described to achieve patient goals with a high level of satisfaction. Gluteal implants, fat transfer, and local tissue rearrangement are the 3 ways to accomplish augmentation and improve contours. Each technique offers unique benefits that are offset by particular risks and limitations. Similar to other areas within plastic surgery, mastery of the craft involves appropriate patient selection and tailoring the operative plan to patient-specific anatomy and desires. An overwhelming amount of interest in the literature relates to female buttock augmentation (also referred to as Brazilian Butt Lift, BBL, S-Curve, and others), because male gluteal augmentation only accounts for approximately 5% to 10% of the gluteal augmentation market in the United States. This article focuses on the latter by emphasizing the nuances of male gluteal contouring and augmentation; particularly, how it differs from the female counterpart.

GENDER-BASED DIFFERENCES IN GLUTEAL ANATOMY

Biologic requirements of pregnancy and childbirth explain the differences between the male and female pelvic structure, which translates to 2 distinct gluteal shapes with vastly different contours. The male pelvis is described as android (heart-shaped), whereas in women, it is gynecoid (rounded-shaped). This is due to differences in average pelvic width, length of sacral bones, and the variable amount of iliac tilt/flare. Men have narrower, shorter pelvic bones with longer sacrums, and parallel iliac bones that do not have much lateral flare. The most superficial muscle in the region, the gluteus maximus, accounts for most of the buttock projection. It originates on the posterior iliac crest, sacral and coccygeal bones and inserts laterally on the greater trochanter. Studies have found that the superficial fascia system is tightly adherent to the periosteum of the iliac crease in men, whereas it is relatively adherent to the muscle fascia in the gluteal depression and several centimeters above the iliac crest in women.[1] These differences are compounded by

[a] Private Practice, Ghavami Plastic Surgery, 433 North Camden Drive, Suite 780, Beverly Hills, CA 90210, USA;
[b] New York Institute of Male Plastic Surgery, 655 Park Avenue, New York, NY 10065, USA
* Corresponding author.
E-mail address: drvranis@gmail.com

Clin Plastic Surg 50 (2023) 615–628
https://doi.org/10.1016/j.cps.2023.05.003
0094-1298/23/© 2023 Elsevier Inc. All rights reserved.

the fact that men tend to have less subcutaneous fat in this region, making the overall shape of the buttock more closely resemble the underlying osseous and muscular contours. The location of fat deposits around the body are influenced by sex chromosomes, hormonal controls, and nutritional input. In men, adipocytes located in the gluteal region and lower body are less efficient at up taking circulating triglyceride–fatty acids from meals, therefore do not hypertrophy as easily compared with female counterparts.[2] These biologic differences contribute to the gender-based phenotypic differences observed in overall body shape, particularly of the gluteal region.

IDEAL MALE GLUTEAL AESTHETICS

The ideal male buttock differs from the female buttock in several ways. Women tend to prefer a round, full buttock with a width that closely approximated the vertical height. A soft, feminine, gentle curve exists as the narrow waist transitions from the midback to the buttock. This has been described to represent an "hourglass." Conversely, a more athletic torso and gluteal silhouette are aesthetically preferred in men. Sharper transitions are expected, as muscles tend to be thicker, and their edges are more evident. This can be seen with the more dramatic lateral gluteal concavity in men. Other abrupt transition points include the latissimus border to the external oblique, as it interdigitates with the thoracolumbar fascia; and from the lower back muscles to the superior aspect of the gluteus maximus. Inferior to the buttock, the hamstrings are well-defined and distinct from the gluteal musculature. In well-developed men, the vertical distance of each gluteus is relatively longer compared with the width and the projection of the buttock and is maintained within the width of the underlying gluteus maximus muscle. This is likely due to the minimal fat content in this region as described above. Projection is equally important to both genders. One commonality between both sexes is that the area of greatest projection should reside in the midpoint of the buttock with a 50:50 vertical ratio above and below this point.

IMPLANT-BASED GLUTEAL AUGMENTATION

The first published record of placing silicone implants in the gluteal region occurred in 1969 when Bartels and colleagues[3] performed the operation to correct unilateral muscular atrophy. Since then, gluteal implants have evolved in design and material. Various sized and anatomic shapes using silicone cohesive and solid elastomer options are now available. These implants have been tried in the subcutaneous, subfascial, intramuscular, and submuscular planes through a single median incision or a double (paramedian) incision technique. Each of these permutations has a unique set of benefits, challenges, and complications. For the most part, subcutaneous implant placement has been abandoned owing to high rates of palpability, migration, malposition, and extrusion. Seasoned surgeons with vast experience with these operations continue to debate ideal incision placement and implant pocket.

In general, the operative sequence is as follows. On the day of surgery, the patient is marked in the standing position, and implant templates are used to template the pocket borders. For both subfascial and intramuscular techniques, the pocket is drawn 2 cm lateral to the sacrum and 5 cm above the infragluteal fold.[4–6] The size or range of sizes considered depends on the patient's height, body habitus, and structural anatomy. Regardless of incision choice (median vs 2 paramedian incisions), dissection begins in the subcutaneous space until the lateral edge of the sacrum is reached. Two centimeters beyond lateral to the sacral border, a 6- to 8-cm fascial incision is made. At that point, a decision is made to elevate a subfascial pocket or continue the dissection to an intermediate depth within the gluteus maximus muscle using electrocautery. If so, typically, 1.5 to 2 cm of muscle coverage is evenly maintained on the superficial aspect of the pocket dissection. Care is taken to avoid inadvertent deep dissection to injure or expose the sciatic nerve. During the dissection, transection of the inferior gluteal nerve is avoided while superior and inferior gluteal artery perforators are controlled with prospective hemostasis with long insulated forceps, if encountered.[7] Also, respecting the lateral border of the gluteus maximus muscle is imperative for 2 reasons: (1) maintains the aesthetically pleasing lateral gluteal concavity and (2) prevents lateral migration of the implant. After the precise pocket dissection, sizers can be used to confirm the extent of pocket dissection and determine the ideal implant volume/dimensions. After implant selection, it is delivered into the pocket followed by a meticulous 5-layer closure (**Fig. 1**). In rare instances, additional customization of implants is warranted. Meticulous shaping of the implant is performed by the surgeon before insertion (**Fig. 2**). Patient education regarding postoperative care (avoiding activities that cause stretching, friction, or pressure to the surgical area) is equally important, as most wound dehiscence complications are thought to be mechanical and occur between days 12 and 16.[8]

A high level of vigilance for maintaining complete sterility minimizes the risk of infection, which is inherently problematic for this operation because of its

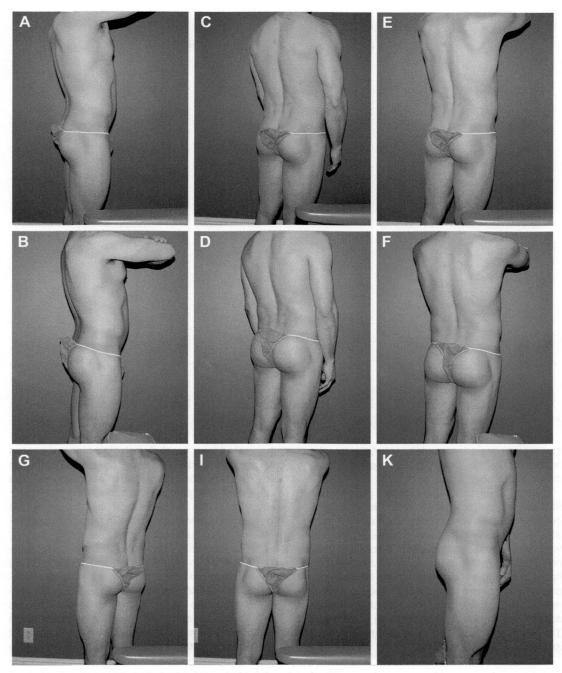

Fig. 1. (*A, C, E, G, I, K, M, O, Q, S, U*) A 32-year-old, 5-foot 9-inch, 170-pound, mesomorphic man underwent intramuscular gluteal implantation with 305-cc custom-contoured silicone implants. (*B, D, F, H, J, L, N, P, R, T, V*) Seventeen months postoperative results demonstrate a natural contour with enhanced gluteal volume, particularly at the superior pole without a visible incision.

proximity to the anus and high rates of wound healing complications. Perioperative precautions to decrease infection risk include appropriate administration of preoperative antibiotics, meticulous preparation/draping, use of antibacterial Ioban drapes to

further isolate the surgical field and prevent skin flora contamination, antibiotic-based pocket irrigation, surgeon glove changes, "no-touch" delivery devices (ie, Keller funnel [Allergan Aesthetics, Irvine, CA]), and a strong watertight closure. If drains are used,

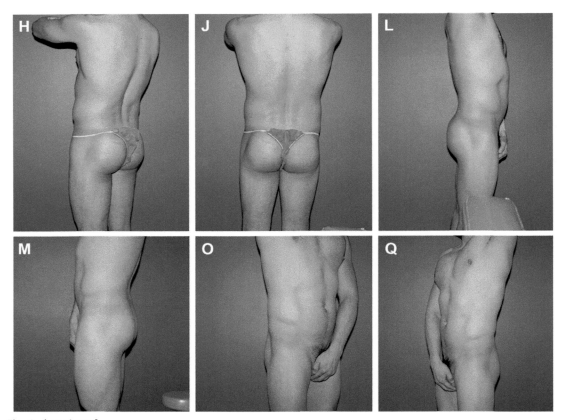

Fig. 1. (*continued*)

some surgeons advocate for continued use of oral antibiotics in the postoperative period until the drains are removed.

Overall, ideal candidates for this procedure are fit, but lack buttock projection. It is important to counsel patients about ptosis if identified preoperatively, as this will not be automatically corrected with the placement of implants. In addition, excess regional adiposity must be evaluated. Ancillary liposuction can be performed at the time of implant placement to refine contours and amplify the appearance of the implant. Selecting the most appropriate implant shape and size is paramount. This involves experience, consideration of regional anatomy, and artistic vision.

GLUTEAL LIPOSCULPTING

Refined torso sculpting from liposuction along with large-volume fat grafting for gluteal augmentation has become significantly more popular for both men and women. This procedure has a smaller incision burden and avoids the inherent risks associated with the implants themselves mentioned above. A major benefit of this procedure is the ability to redistribute the location of the fat cells. Fat is

harvested from carefully selected areas of excess to highlight underlying skeletomuscular definition (ie, rectus abdominus, external obliques, serratus anterior interdigitations, deltoids, pectoralis major muscles). This is performed by debulking the deep layer (ie, subscarpal fat in the abdomen) followed by careful sculpting the superficial layer (ie, suprascarpal fat). Liposuction of the flanks narrows the width of the waist and thereby alters the waist-to-hip ratio even before the surgeon embarks on the buttock portion of the procedure. By decreasing the thickness of the subcutaneous layer and accentuating the shadows between various anatomic muscular-skeletal transitions of the abdomen, flanks, chest, and arms, desirable athletic definition can be unveiled. After the fat is collected, processed, and prepared for injection, the surgeon artistically delivers the fat to shape the gluteal region. Adherence to previously described fat-grafting principles in order to optimize graft survival includes delicate processing of fat, injection with low sheer-force devices, and avoidance of overgrafting. Ultimately, the goal is to create an aesthetically pleasing buttock with masculine characteristics that is balanced with the rest of the torso and legs.

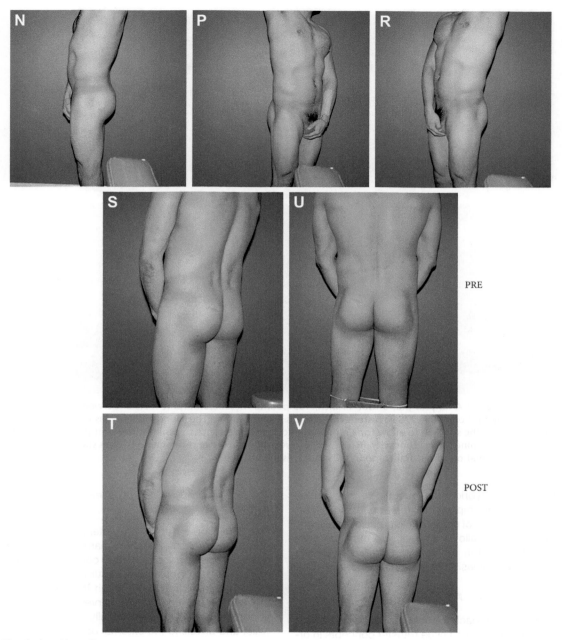

Fig. 1. (continued)

Most men desire highlighting gluteal musculature, mimicking the shape of a well-trained athlete. Thus, fat is delivered preferentially to the superior and inferior poles of the buttock, creating an elongated aesthetically masculine appearance. Oftentimes, the superior and inferior poles need to be widened as well as augmented. Medial and central projection enhances the appearance of the gluteus maximus and gives the illusion of a taller buttock. Judicious amounts of fat, if any, are placed in the midlateral region. It is critical to avoid lateral expansion, which will have a rounding effect on the buttock. As mentioned previously in the article, the ideal male gluteal aesthetic is a more oblong shape with a greater height-to-width ratio. Meticulous technical skill is required to prevent the creation of sharp corners and a rectangular shelf, as this appears unnatural.

In addition, fat transfer can be used to fine-tune gluteal contours after placement of a gluteal

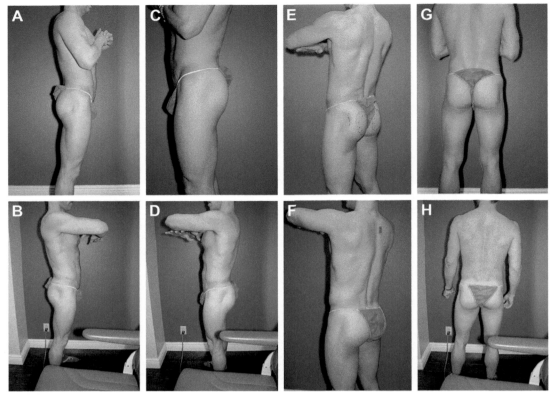

Fig. 2. (*A, C, E, G*) A 42-year-old, 5-foot 11-inch, 165-pound, mesoectomorphic man underwent intramuscular gluteal augmentation with a 276-cc custom-contoured silicone implant. The round implant was trimmed medially and laterally by the surgeon to allow for a more athletic, lean appearance to achieve sufficient posterior convexity while maintaining lateral concavity. (*B, D, F, H*) Five-year postoperative result demonstrates stability in volume increases preservation of natural contours without a visible incision.

implant. This hybrid technique allows the surgeon to camouflage implant borders, softening transitions from areas of convexity to areas of concavity. This ultimately allows surgeons to maintain even greater control in the operating room to deliver aesthetically pleasing contours (**Figs. 3** and **4**).

MALE GLUTEAL AUTOAUGMENTATION

A modern approach to male gluteal augmentation involves harnessing tissue transfer concepts in order to repurpose adjacent tissue for improvements in buttock projection and create an aesthetically pleasing male buttock overall. Although powerful in simultaneously transforming the shape of the waist and buttock, gluteal autoaugmentation procedures can only be offered to a narrow patient population.[9] Typically, patients with massive weight loss present with excess adiposity and skin laxity of the anterior and posterior torso. Those who are willing to accept the well-hidden circumferential scar burden are considered good candidates for this procedure.

The 360° Torso Tuck with Gluteal "Wallet Flap" Autoaugmentation

The 360° Torso Tuck with gluteal "Wallet Flap" Autoaugmentation procedure harnesses multiple plastic surgery principles and concepts to ultimately create a balanced, natural, aesthetically pleasing athletic result. Although the patient is in the supine position, fat is harvested from the abdomen and flanks, essentially narrowing the waist and unveiling the external oblique musculature, inferior ribs, and iliac crest without compromising blood supply to the abdominoplasty flap. The patient is carefully turned and secured in the prone position. Using pinch-and-displacement techniques, preoperative markings are confirmed on the table. The width and height of the "wallet flap" as well as the associated pocket dimensions have also been previously marked based on the patient's anatomy. The pocket is envisioned with bias toward the medial aspect of the buttock. This ensures that the medial and central regions of the buttock will be augmented over the gluteus

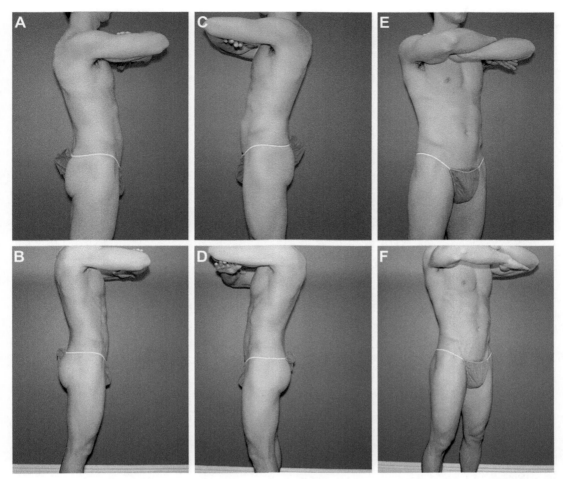

Fig. 3. (*A, C, E, G, H, I, M, O, Q, S, U, W, Y*) This 29-year-old, 5-foot 11-inch, 165-pound, ectomorphic athlete underwent intramuscular gluteal augmentation with a 276-cc custom-contoured silicone implant. BodyBanking fat transfer was performed to add additional volume superiorly. The hybrid technique allowed for shape customization, elongating the appearance of the gluteal musculature and preventing implant visibility and an artificial appearance. (*B, D, F, H, J, K, L, N, P, R, T, V, X, Z*) Twenty-one-month postoperative results demonstrating natural contours, increased volume, and enhanced shape without a visible incision.

maximus muscle without widening or rounding the buttock shape. After incisions are made, an inferiorly based oblong flap is developed on each side. The deep dissection is carried inferiorly in the subfascial plane to allow for reflection of the flap. A deep subcutaneous pocket is created within the inferior gluteal flap using the exact dimensions of the flap. This concept is analogous to the precise creation of a pocket, allowing for the placement of a gluteal implant. The flap is folded over itself, in the superioinferior trajectory, and secured into the previously created custom pocket ensuring not to compromise blood supply. The inferior gluteal flap is translated superiorly and meticulously reapproximated to the superior back flap for closure. Lateral dog ears are dealt with after

the patient returns to the supine position and the abdominoplasty portion of the procedure is performed. Supplemental fat grafting (or BodyBanking, as described by the senior author) can be used on the posterior or anterior side to fine tune shape and enhance contours.

DISCUSSION

Many differences exist between the 2 sexes with regards to gluteal cosmetic surgery (**Table 1**). The innate structural differences between the android and gynecoid pelvis represent the foundation and major underlying contribution to the buttock shape and contour. Furthermore, differences in muscle mass and regional fat deposition

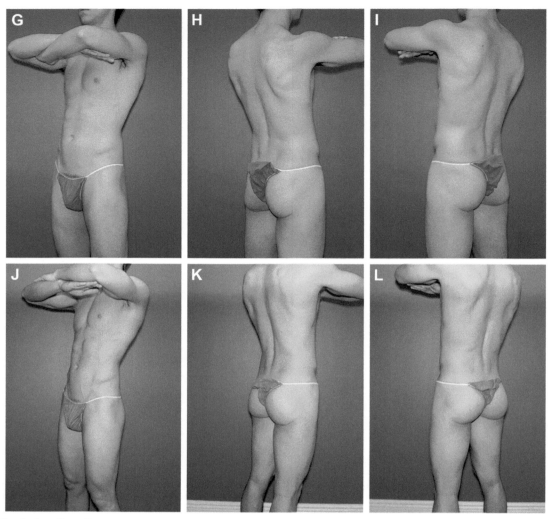

Fig. 3. (*continued*)

have been described in the literature. Preoperative observation classifies men into 3 categories based on height, baseline muscle mass, and fat deposition: endomorph, mesomorph, and ecto-morph. Oftentimes the excess skin obscures underlying muscle tone and contours, but it is important to appreciate which category a patient belongs to.

Society and culture influence aesthetic ideals, which guide the surgeon to artistically sculpt an aesthetically pleasing buttock. To do so, a plastic surgeon relies on various techniques and plastic surgery principles to accomplish this task. When performing body modification and body contouring procedures, it is important to create balance and harmony among the anterior/posterior torso and gluteal definition. A highly sculpted buttock and posterior torso would look strange on a patient with an obese abdomen and wide thighs that lack definition. Although this article focuses on gluteal augmentation and shaping, it touches on other regional anatomic areas, as these procedures typically complement each other and improve the overall aesthetic result.

Gluteal Implants

Gluteal implant surgery can produce remarkable results with significant improvements in projection, volume, and shape. However, it also carries high rates of complications, up to 38%, reported in a multicenter survey published a decade ago.[7] Since then, surgeons have consciously implemented various modifications in their practice to decrease complications. Many surgeons advocate for separate incisions for each implant instead of a median

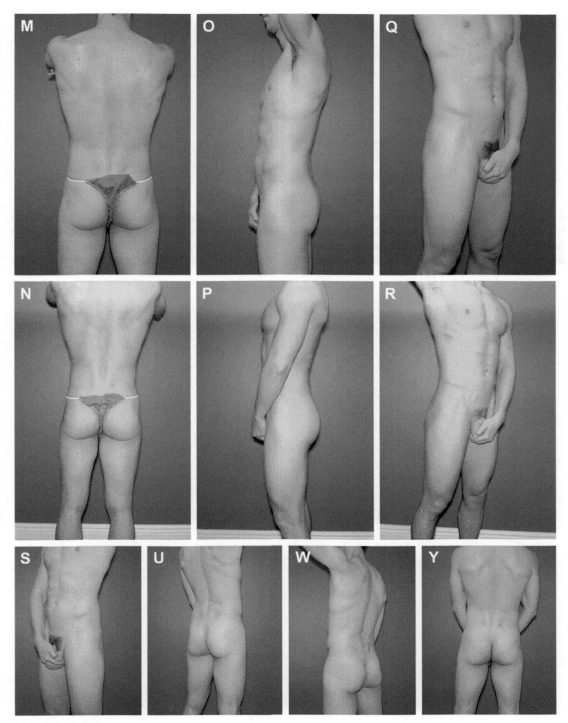

Fig. 3. (*continued*)

incision over the sacrum—which decreased the rate of wound dehiscence rates from 30% to 5% in one practice.[8] The senior author also endorses that a low complication rate can be achieved through 2 paramedian incisions when the implants are placed intramuscularly, and certain intraoperative precautions described above are implemented. Ultimately, these procedural modifications require

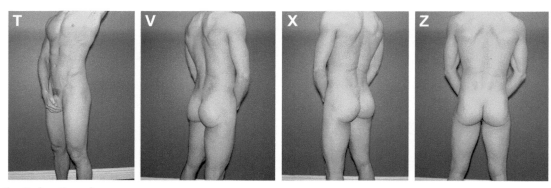

Fig. 3. (*continued*)

further investigation to determine their contribution to minimizing complications while maintaining aesthetic outcomes. There are certain benefits and drawbacks with each pocket plane selection.

Both the subfascial and the intramuscular pockets offer good implant coverage. When placed within the muscle, the implant is less palpable and has a lower rate of migration. This is due to the greater

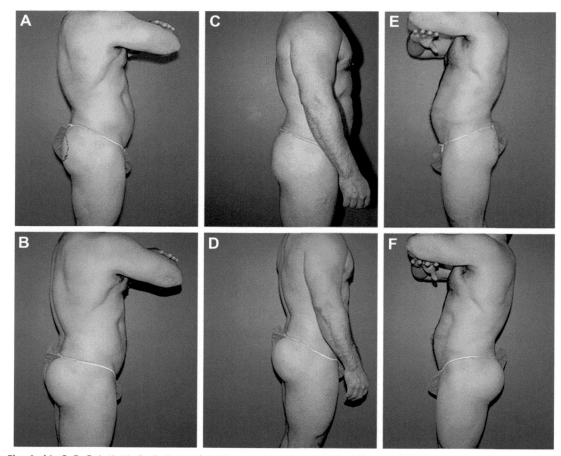

Fig. 4. (*A, C, E, G, I, K, M, O, Q, S, U, W*) A 46-year-old, 5-foot 7-inch, 168-pound, endomesomorphic man underwent intramuscular gluteal implantation with a 330-cc custom-contoured silicone implant. BodyBanking principles were used to harvest fat from the flanks and transfer to the superior aspect of the buttocks. (*B, D, F, H, J, L, N, P, R, T, V, X*) The composite technique resulted in a more elongated, muscular appearance. Thirty-five-month postoperative results demonstrate a well-maintained natural contour and enhanced superior gluteal volume without a visible incision.

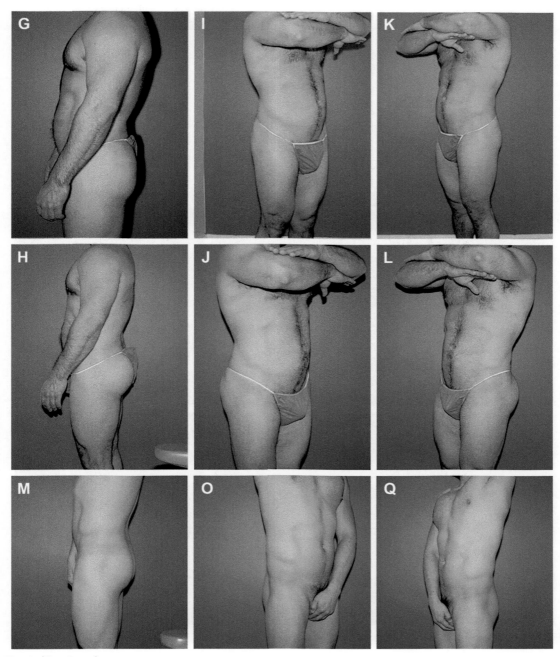

Fig. 4. (*Continued*)

amount of padding; however, there is a theoretical risk of sciatic nerve compression given its proximity to deeper structures.

Gluteal Fat Transfer

Fat grafting has gained popularity, as this procedure avoids the longer incisions required for implant-based gluteal contouring that can result in high rates of dehiscence along with the inherent risks associated with the implants themselves—malposition, migration, palpability, and infection. Various techniques with regard to collecting, separating, processing, and delivering the fat have been described; however, that discussion is outside the scope of this article.

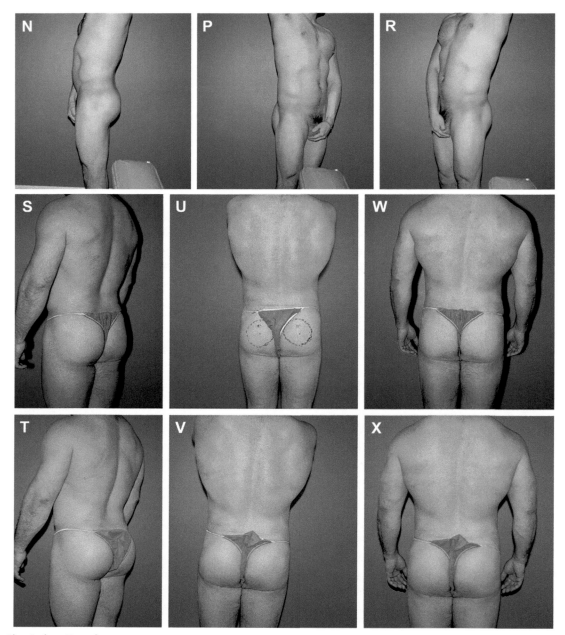

Fig. 4. (*continued*)

The fat harvest portion of the procedure presents an opportunity for the surgeon to debulk and sculpt distant and nearby donor areas. These changes affect the shape of the entire torso, not just the buttock. In fact, they often enhance the appearance of the buttock, as the surgeon is able to create harmony between the adjacent anatomic areas. However, a potential downfall of fat transfer is that as the patient's weight fluctuates, the size and shape will mirror these fluctuations and perhaps lose the aesthetic appeal created at the time of surgery.

Additional limitations to this procedure must be considered. Thin patients that lack an adequate amount of adiposity from all donor sites are not candidates for this procedure or might be better suited for a hybrid procedure (implant and fat transfer). The inherent uncertainty of fat graft

Table 1
Differences and considerations between male and female buttock augmentation

	Male	Female
Gluteal/pelvic anatomy	• Thicker gluteal fascia • Less body fat stored, greater bone and muscle mass • Android pelvis (heart-shaped) • Narrower pelvic bones • Longer and narrower sacrum	• Wider angle of iliac crest tilt • More body fat stored • Gynecoid pelvis (rounded shape) • Wider pelvic bones
Aesthetic ideals of the buttock	• Athletic appearance • Well-defined lateral gluteal concavity • Greater height-to-width ratio • Waist-to-hip ratio approximates 0.9	• Round and voluptuous • Soft lateral gluteal concavity or mild convexity • Wider • Waist-to-hip ratio approximates 0.6
Implant characteristics	• Smaller • Round	• Larger • Anatomic
Autoaugmentation procedures	• Vertical turnover flap ("wallet flap")	• Rotational flap (lateral to inferior rotation)

viability after transfer is a consideration. Current estimates predict that 70% to 80% of the fat transferred will survive.[10,11] Thus, surgeons will "overcorrect" knowing that there will be a certain amount of "deflation" that occurs within the first 6 to 9 months, even if a patient's weight remains constant. The senior surgeon strongly advocates for a high carbohydrate diet in the postoperative period to encourage graft survival and implantation. Even after attempting to optimize all of the known variables, unlike implant-based gluteal augmentation whereby the shape and volume of the implant will remain constant, a small amount of unpredictable change in shape and volume will take place from the on-table result to the long-term result with fat-grafting procedures. This reality can be bothersome to both the surgeon and the patient, particularly as the patients get used to the size/shape immediately after surgery when edema and the volume transferred are at their greatest.

Last, numerous cases of fat embolus and death have been reported as a consequence of large-volume fat grafting to the gluteal region. The risk of fat embolus can be mitigated by grafting in the subcutaneous plane and taking the necessary precautions that involve patient positioning, use of large-bore stiff cannulas, and calculated incision placement for ideal cannula angulation to avoid piercing the deep fascia. To date, very few surgeons prefer intramuscular fat injection advocating for the ability to harness greater projection.[12,13] However, caution must be maintained when using this technique, as the risk for big vessel injury, fat migration, and fat embolus increases with these maneuvers.

Gluteal Autoaugmentation

In the appropriate candidate, the "wallet flap" autoaugmentation procedure yields excellent aesthetic results. The design of the flap with a vertical turnover from the superior to inferior direction preferentially adds volume to the superiomedial aspect of the buttock. The bulk created by folding tissue over itself ultimately creates a prominent, athletic-appearing superior gluteal crease. Medial bias in pocket design avoids unnecessary excess volume laterally, which ultimately translates to a more masculine oblong gluteal shape. The amount of additional inferior pole volume that can be achieved from the flap depends on how much tissue laxity the patient presents. This is determined by the distance between the upper and lower incision lines, which approximates the amount of turnover one can expect from the flap. Fortunately, by lifting the inferior gluteal skin over the "wallet flap," the inferior gluteal crease becomes more defined. The redraping of redundant skin also contributes to a more youthful, taut, rejuvenated appearance. Additional inferior pole volume can be added through the use of fat-grafting/BodyBanking techniques. The vertical fold-over "wallet flap" autoaugmentation differs from other rotational autoaugmentation techniques that have been described in the literature for body lift procedures in patients with massive weight loss. Those procedures rotate superiolateral tissue to the central aspect of the buttock, but the bulk from the rotation point remains in the superior lateral quadrant, which is less than ideal in male gluteal aesthetics.

CLINICS CARE POINTS

- Regardless of technique, the goal is to augment medial and central projection (superiorly and inferiorly) to maintain a narrowed, muscular-appearing buttock with a dramatic lateral gluteal concavity.
- Evaluation should include the entire torso, buttock, and thighs. Ancillary procedures, such as liposculpting and fat transfer/Body-Banking, should be considered to enhance the overall aesthetic result.
- Creating harmony and balance between the buttock and nearby anatomic areas is critical in attaining a natural-appearing buttock.
- Preservation of the trochanteric depression along with dramatic highlights of the gluteal musculature is critical to deliver an athletic, aesthetically pleasing male buttock.
- Postoperative high carbohydrate diet is critical for fat graft survival and minimizing complications while maintaining consistency in long-term results.

Pitfalls

- Gluteal implants are associated with high complication rates; adherence to important preoperative, intraoperative, and postoperative considerations to maintain sterility and prevent wound dehiscence greatly decreases complication rates.
- Meticulous intramuscular dissection avoids inadvertent damage to deep structures (ie, sciatic nerve).

DISCLOSURE

Dr N.M. Vranis does not have any financial or commercial disclosures relevant to this article. Dr D. Steinbrech receives book royalties from Thieme and Elsevier; in addition, has financial investment in Allergan Aesthetics (AbbVie) and Alpha Aesthetics.

REFERENCES

1. Lockwood TE. Superficial fascial system (SFS) of the trunk and extremities: a new concept. Plast Reconstr Surg 1991;87:1009–18.
2. Fried SK, Lee MJ, Karastergiou K. Shaping fat distribution: new insights into the molecular determinants of depot- and sex-dependent adipose biology. Obesity 2015;23(7):1345–52.
3. Bartels RJ, O'Malley JE, Douglas WM, et al. An unusual use of the Cronin breast prosthesis. Case report. Plast Reconstr Surg 1969;44(5):500.
4. de la Pena JA. Subfascial technique for gluteal augmentation. Aesthetic Surg J 2004;24(3):265–73.
5. Salibian AA, Steinbrech DS. Intramuscular gluteal augmentation with silicone implant. In: Steinbrech DS, editor. Male aesthetic plastic surgery. 1st Ed. New York, NY: Thieme; 2021. p. 473–96.
6. Steinbrech DS, Gonzalez E. Male gluteal augmentation with BodyBankingTM Lipocell transfer and silicone implant. In: Cansancao AL, Conde-Green A, editors. Gluteal fat augmentation: best practices in brazilian butt lift. 1st Ed. Switzerland: Springer; 2021. p. 199–211.
7. Mofid NM, Gonzalez R, de la Pena JA, et al. Buttock Augmentation with silicone implants: a multicenter survey review of 2226 patients. Plast Reconstr Surg 2013;131(4):897–901.
8. de la Pena JA, Gallardo G. Subfascial male buttock augmentation. In: Steinbrech DS, editor. Male aesthetic plastic surgery. 1st Ed. New York, NY: Thieme; 2021. p. 463–72.
9. Steinbrech DS, Piazza RC. 360o torso tuck with gluteal "wallet flap" autoaugmentation. In: Steinbrech DS, editor. Male aesthetic plastic surgery. 1st Ed. New York, NY: Thieme; 2021. p. 363–76.
10. Sinno S, Wilson S, Brownstone N, et al. Current thoughts on fat grafting: using the evidence to determine fact or fiction. Plast Reconstr Surg 2016;137(3):818–24.
11. Abboud MH, Dibo SA, Abboud NM. Power-assisted gluteal augmentation: a new technique for sculpting, harvesting and transferring fat. Aesthetic Surg J 2015;35(8):987–94.
12. Mendieta CG. Gluteal reshaping. Aesthetic Surg J 2007;27(6):641–55.
13. Mendieta C. The art of gluteal sculpting. 1st ed. New York, NY: Thieme; 2011.

Art and Safety of Gluteal Augmentation
Future Directions

David M. Stepien, MD, PhD[a], Ashkan Ghavami, MD[b,c],*

KEYWORDS

- Safety • Aesthetic education • Technology • Tissue engineering • Radiofrequency • Ultrasound
- Artificial intelligence • Gluteal fat transfer

KEY POINTS

- Safety measures including ultrasound and smart cannulas can increase safety in gluteal augmentation.
- Education in safe gluteal augmentation will be critical in residency and fellowship programs.
- Advancements in technology offer methods of improving surgical planning, soft tissue management, and tissue engineering.

INTRODUCTION

Gluteal augmentation, more than any other aesthetic procedure, has undergone remarkable advancement and controversies over the past 20 years. The transition from implants to autologous fat transfer techniques began a rapid evolution of the entire practice of gluteal augmentation. Autologous fat grafting offers a more controlled, personalized, long-term functional, and natural result while addressing surrounding anatomical regions that define the buttock shape, making this procedure a superior approach compared to gluteal implants alone.[1] This advance was accompanied by a rise in social media and public desire for buttock augmentation.[2,3] Innovative surgeons saw the potential for social media in reaching a far wider audience in terms of marketing while also removing stigma and secrecy from plastic surgery. This opened the proverbial floodgates in terms of new gluteal augmentation patients; however, with the meteoric growth of gluteal augmentation we also saw a rise in complications specific to this approach. Rightfully, mortality associated with fat embolism brought about intense scrutiny related to the safety of gluteal augmentation with autologous fat.[4] Through the collaboration of the major societies in plastic surgery (ISAPS, ASAPS, ASPS, ASERF), clear guidelines were constructed to markedly improve the safety of this procedure and protect the future of autologous fat grafting for gluteal augmentation.[5] A positive consequence of this collaboration so early in the development of an aesthetic procedure is the culture of innovation around gluteal augmentation and in its education.[6] This has been championed by the premier figures of the aesthetic plastic surgery community and continues to foster new pathways for innovation in gluteal augmentation.[7] Continuing this evolution will be key in advancing our field as plastic surgeons, and importantly, to safely deliver better outcomes for our patients. In this article, we examine the future of gluteal augmentation through the categories of safety, education, and technology.

[a] Duke Plastic Surgery, 2301 Erwin Road, Durham, NC 27710, USA; [b] Division of Plastic Surgery, David Geffen UCLA School of Medicine, UCLA Plastic Surgery, 200 Medcal Plaza Driveway, Suite 460, Los Angeles, CA 90095, USA; [c] Private Practice, Ghavami Plastic Surgery, Inc., 433 North Camden Drive, Suite 780, Beverly Hills, CA 90210, USA
* Corresponding author. Ghavami Plastic Surgery, 433 North Camden Drive, Suite 780, Beverly Hills, CA 90210.
E-mail address: ashghavami@yahoo.com

Clin Plastic Surg 50 (2023) 629–633
https://doi.org/10.1016/j.cps.2023.06.009

SAFETY

The crux of safety in gluteal fat transfer is not different than any other surgical endeavor in history, and that is *education*. This is an operation that is largely ignored in residency training programs and most aesthetic fellowships in the United States, to the point where residents and recent graduates are seeking out private practice surgeons in the US and abroad to learn from. It is the senior author's contention that any and all future directions in advancing the specialty of gluteal augmentation with fat (as well as accompanying body contouring) must start here. Due to this lack of education and formal training, safety has become the primary driver in advancing the field of gluteal augmentation. From the tumultuous early era of this procedure to its current status as a widely practiced and safe operation, great strides have been made.[8] Continued dedication to safety in gluteal augmentation will continue to be at the forefront of future innovation. Early improvements in safety were achieved through task force work to identify the anatomical considerations leading to fat embolization.[4] This lead to the recommendations for entirely subcutaneous augmentation and avoiding intramuscular injection of fat.[7] To continue improving the safety of this procedure, standardizing techniques to avoid intramuscular or "danger zone" injection is paramount.[9]

Recent recommendations have encouraged the routine use of intra-operative ultrasound to clearly identify the planes of injection as well as vascular anatomy around the injection cannula.[6] This has been introduced quite successfully into routine practice with the Aesthetic Society recommending ultrasound be used for all gluteal fat augmentation and the state of Florida mandating its use in all cases.[10] While many surgeons are already comfortable with using ultrasound as a common modality, there will remain a barrier to access of ultrasound in many private offices and centers. Expanded access to ultrasound training and equipment will aid in further disseminating the utility of ultrasound in gluteal augmentation. However, using ultrasound while moving a canula with a high excursion stroke count is a challenge and techniques have been espoused that rely on "bolus" type injection which have been largely discouraged in the past for increasing the possibility of fat necrosis or "blow out" problems.[11]

Integration of so-called "smart cannulas" also offers a potential new pathway for safety in gluteal augmentation. Turer and co-workers have developed a detachable unit that integrates with current cannula systems to sense electrical impedance by surrounding tissues during fat injection.[12] Electrical impedance, the opposition to alternating current, is much lower in muscle than fat as muscle tissue has lower resistance to electrical current. While the cannula is in contact with adipose tissue in the subcutaneous plane, impedance will be relatively high and injection of fat will continue normally. If the cannula enters muscle, however, the impedance will drop significantly. At a far higher speed than human tactile detection, the cannula will sense the change and immediately disable injection of fat until the cannula is withdrawn from muscle tissue. This simple yet effective system may allow a method for standardizing the plane of injection and further improve safety for patients undergoing gluteal fat grafting.

EDUCATION

As mentioned above, educational outreach has been a necessary default to the paucity in more structured educational systems. All this is to improving safety as well as aesthetic outcomes on gluteal augmentation, as it would be for other aesthetic surgeries. Once a somewhat niche practice relegated to a few innovative practitioners, gluteal augmentation panels are present at essentially every major plastic surgery society meeting. In fact, the senior author clearly remembers the first ever Gluteal Augmentation Panel at the Annual ASAPS Meeting in San Francisco in which he was a panelist. At that time focus was largely on concepts and techniques. Currently, cadaver courses and live surgery programs have become increasingly popular and offer instruction to a broad audience. This tends, however, to target the post-training demographic with those already in practice and familiar with aesthetic surgical approaches. While important, education for practitioners at this level often leaves out foundational information for those without the same aesthetic surgical skill level and particularly surgical trainees.

Plastic surgery residency programs have demonstrated a definite shift in recent years toward a desire for more aesthetic surgery training.[13] The nature of most academic program environments within a hospital-based practice limits trainee access to aesthetic surgery and heavily emphasizes reconstructive procedures.[14] With the inclusion of select aesthetic procedures in the mandatory case minimums for graduation in US plastic surgery residency programs, graduating senior residents are often left scrambling to meet their aesthetic surgery minimums prior to the completion of training. While the traditional solution has been academic programs partnering with community private practice groups to gain aesthetic exposure, high-level programs are beginning to recruit plastic surgeons to develop aesthetic surgery practices within the academic group.[14] This serves to greatly enhance resident aesthetic education as well as offering increased revenue for the academic department. For the aesthetic community, this offers the power of academic institution resources for research and development in aesthetic surgery. This new environment allows the introduction of education on safe and effective gluteal augmentation at the resident training level.

This is further refined with the expansion of resident aesthetic surgery clinics where senior residents under the supervision of an attending surgeon can perform their own aesthetic procedures often at significantly reduced cost for patients.[15] Integration of gluteal augmentation into chief resident clinics presents a hands-on opportunity for residents to practice safe surgical technique and maximize their educational impact. This also puts more patients under the care of board eligible and certified plastic surgeons and ultimately will continue to improve the safety profile in gluteal augmentation.

With the popularity of aesthetic surgery fellowships increasing year by year, mandating education in gluteal augmentation in fellowship also presents an opportunity for further refining training. Aesthetic surgery fellows have the opportunity to assist in gluteal augmentation cases with their fellowship faculty as well as performing their own cases in fellowship-sponsored fellows' clinics. An interesting opportunity arises to offer certification in autologous fat gluteal augmentation similar to the subspecialty certificate (formerly certificate of added qualification CAQ) in surgery of the hand. This could be through the completion of a specified fellowship curriculum, case minimums, or societal review. This certification program could serve to demonstrate safety as well as provide assurance for hospital systems or surgery centers that a surgeon has demonstrated safety and experience in gluteal fat transfer techniques.

Through a variety of mechanisms, the future of gluteal augmentation will rely on improvement in education to allow both safe conduct of these surgeries by new surgeons and continued development in the field through new surgical innovators inspired by their exposure during residency and fellowship.

TECHNOLOGY

Technological advancements in aesthetic surgery present unique opportunities for improving outcomes. Gluteal fat transfer falls at the intersection of several areas of technological advancement in the short and long term. Through exploring each application, we can begin to anticipate the future trajectory of gluteal augmentation.

Radiofrequency Technologies

Among the most important new technologies in body contouring, radiofrequency technology has clearly demonstrated itself as a front-runner in this space. Radiofrequency allows simultaneous management of the quality and laxity of skin at the time of liposuction and body contouring excisional procedures.[16] Previously, liposuction results were limited by resultant skin laxity. With the addition of radiofrequency skin tightening, we have been able to push the limits of liposculpting while creating excellent outcomes at the skin level. This has multiple potential applications in gluteal fat transfer as a modality for the treatment of both the donor and recipient sites. The InMode Bodytite and Morpheus systems and Renuvion J-plasma have become common adjuncts to our body contouring practices.[17] Frequently we treat both the superficial skin with Morpheus and the deeper dermis and subcutaneous layer with BodyTite or Renuvion at the time of liposuction.[17] These can also be used in the buttock to achieve skin tightening prior to grafting so as to avoid overfilling to overcome skin laxity. In revisional surgery such as reversal procedures, these technologies will have forefront role to improve buttock contour in the setting of significant tissue debulking. Significant work will need to be done in terms of characterizing the improvement in outcomes with the addition of these technologies and understanding their effects on grafted fat but they offer an exciting opportunity for investigation in gluteal augmentation surgery.

Artificial Intelligence

Artificial intelligence (AI) technology has had a meteoric rise in recent years. Openly available AI platforms have been used to analyze massive amounts of data to produce images, videos, and text at increasingly impressive qualities.[18] With this ability to incorporate an almost infinite amount of data, AI presents an opportunity to improve gluteal augmentation through surgical planning, patient communication, and improving consistency. While very little early work has been done bringing AI into surgical planning, the potential is clear. Through collaboration with data scientists and AI platforms, vast databases of patient images can be analyzed, and the AI systems trained to identify potential outcomes as well as specific interventions that can be used to achieve them. In conjunction with a well-trained surgeon, AI can augment the pre-operative analysis process and optimize the planned gluteal augmentation to direct the areas of augmentation. AI can also generate images of potential outcomes based on a patient baseline anatomy to enhance pre and postoperative communication with patients by showing them what is possible to achieve with their anatomy. This predictive imaging can be further developed for use in the OR where specific areas can be identified using AI and panned filled volumes can be suggested. None of this will replace surgical skill or human evaluation but when used by a well-trained surgeon, AI can be a potential force multiplier for gluteal augmentation outcomes.

Tissue Engineering

Basic science advancements have been fueled by the roles of fat grafting particularly in regenerative medicine and reconstructive surgery.[19] This has allowed for improved access to funding sources for translational scientists studying fat grafting and the cellular biology around it. The aesthetic surgery community will also benefit from advancement in tissue engineering as the application of tissue engineering in elective aesthetic surgery will open entirely new avenues for surgical enhancement. One of the growing aspects of tissue engineering is adipose tissue. In contrast to more highly specialized tissues (organs, muscle, nerve) fat is relatively simplistic in its components.[20] An acellular stromal framework supports adipocytes and allows the vascularization of a largely static tissue. The stem cells that become adipocytes can be isolated and introduced into an appropriate matrix and cultivated to form adipose tissue.[21] As our ability to upscale this engineering improves, it is entirely feasible that we will be able to submit samples of a patient's adipose tissue for cultivation into fat suitable for grafting. This would obviate the need for donor sites and create an essentially infinite source for fat useful in all aspects of regenerative medicine including gluteal augmentation. Even more proximal to this tissue-in-a-flask future is enhanced fat graft take through molecular optimization.[22] These modalities will be integrated into aesthetic surgery as they emerge and offer new opportunities for enhancing our outcomes.

SUMMARY

Gluteal augmentation has arrived at a time in plastic surgery where we have our greatest reach for new patients and interest in aesthetic surgery has reached an all-time high. Within this same climate comes the easy media (social media) propagation of the unfortunate morbidity and mortality that has become linked to gluteal fat transfer and the "BBL" fervor. It is imperative that education in anatomy, pre-operative evaluation, concepts, and safe technical execution becomes systematic and widespread. With surgeons confidently creating great outcomes using safe, consistent, and reproducibly safe techniques, it is tempting to become complacent in the development of this field. However, with so many new technologies and opportunities for growth, gluteal augmentation offers a unique opportunity for further development that more established procedures lack. The incorporation of advances in safety, education, and technology will carry gluteal augmentation into entirely new realms of innovation that can serve to guide aesthetic surgery beyond the single surgeon technique or case series realm and into the forefront of aesthetic surgery evolution.

DISCLOSURE

Dr D.M. Stepien has no relevant disclosures. Dr A. Ghavami: Royalties Thieme Pub, QMP, and Consultant/Advisor for MTF Inc, Advisor/Marketing Partner Inmode, Inc.

REFERENCES

1. Ghavami A. Commentary: gluteal augmentation with silicone implants: a new proposal for intramuscular dissection. Aesthetic Plast Surg 2017;41(5):1148–9.
2. . American Society of Plastic Surgeons. ASPS national clearinghouse of plastic surgery procedural statistics. Plastic Surgery Statistics Report 2018; 1–8.
3. . American Society of Plastic Surgeons. ASPS national clearinghouse of plastic surgery procedural statistics. Plastic Surgery Statistics Report 2020; 1–7.
4. Mofid MM, Teitelbaum S, Suissa D, et al. Report on mortality from gluteal fat grafting: recommendations from the ASERF Task force. Aesthet Surg J 2017; 37(7):796–806.
5. Rubin JP, Walden JL, Lee BT, et al. Statement on patient safety during gluteal fat grafting endorsed by the international society for aesthetic plastic surgery (ISAPS), American society of plastic surgeons (ASPS), the aesthetic society, the plastic surgery foundation (PSF), the aesthetic surgery education and research foundation (ASERF), the international society of plastic regenerative surgeons (ISPRES), the international federation for adipose therapeutics

and science (IFATS) and. Aesthetic Plast Surg 2023; 47(2):894–6.

6. Del Vecchio D, Kenkel JM. Practice advisory on gluteal fat grafting. Aesthet Surg J 2022;42(9): 1019–29.

7. Villanueva NL, Del Vecchio DA, Afrooz PN, et al. Staying safe during gluteal fat transplantation. Plast Reconstr Surg 2018;141(1):79–86.

8. Rios L, Gupta V. Improvement in brazilian butt lift (BBL) safety with the current recommendations from ASERF, ASAPS, and ISAPS. Aesthet Surg J 2020;40(8):864–70.

9. Ghavami A, Villanueva NL, Amirlak B. Gluteal ligamentous anatomy and its implication in safe buttock augmentation. Plast Reconstr Surg 2018;142(2): 363–71.

10. Cansancao AL, Conde-Green A, Vidigal RA, et al. Real-time ultrasound-assisted gluteal fat grafting. Plast Reconstr Surg 2018;142(2):372–6.

11. Ghavami A. Discussion: clinical implications of gluteal fat graft migration: a dynamic anatomical study. Plast Reconstr Surg 2018;142(5):1193–5.

12. Turer DM, Qaium EB, Lawrence AM, et al. A smart sensing cannula for fat grafting. Plast Reconstr Surg 2019;144(2):385–8.

13. Morris MP, Toyoda Y, Christopher AN, et al. A systematic review of aesthetic surgery training within plastic surgery training programs in the USA: an in-depth analysis and practical reference. Aesthetic Plast Surg 2022;46(1):513–23.

14. Perdikis G, Eaves FF, Glassman GE, et al. Aesthetic surgery in plastic surgery academia. Aesthet Surg J 2021;41(7):829–41.

15. Chen J, Lee E, El Eter L, et al. A systematic review on the implementation and educational value of resident aesthetic clinics. Ann Plast Surg 2022;89(2): 152–8.

16. Theodorou SJ, Del Vecchio D, Chia CT. Soft tissue contraction in body contouring with radiofrequency-assisted liposuction: a treatment gap solution. Aesthet Surg J 2018;38(suppl_2):S74–83.

17. Dayan E, Chia C, Burns AJ, et al. Adjustable depth fractional radiofrequency combined with bipolar radiofrequency: a minimally invasive combination treatment for skin laxity. Aesthet Surg J 2019; 39(Suppl_3):S112–9.

18. Liang X, Yang X, Yin S, et al. Artificial intelligence in plastic surgery: applications and challenges. Aesthetic Plast Surg 2021;45(2):784–90.

19. Stosich MS, Mao JJ. Adipose tissue engineering from human adult stem cells: clinical implications in plastic and reconstructive surgery. Plast Reconstr Surg 2007;119(1):71–83.

20. Debels H, Palmer J, Han XL, et al. In vivo tissue engineering of an adipose tissue flap using fat grafts and Adipogel. J Tissue Eng Regen Med 2020; 14(4):633–44.

21.. Assad H, Assad A, Kumar A. Recent developments in 3D bio-printing and its biomedical applications. Pharmaceutics 2023;15(1):1–45.

22. Volz AC, Huber B, Kluger PJ. Adipose-derived stem cell differentiation as a basic tool for vascularized adipose tissue engineering. Differentiation 2016; 92(1–2):52–64.

UNITED STATES POSTAL SERVICE ®

Statement of Ownership, Management, and Circulation
(All Periodicals Publications Except Requester Publications)

1. Publication Title	2. Publication Number	3. Filing Date
CLINICS IN PLASTIC SURGERY	006 – 530	9/18/2023

4. Issue Frequency	5. Number of Issues Published Annually	6. Annual Subscription Price
JAN, APR, JUL,OCT	4	$559.00

7. Complete Mailing Address of Known Office of Publication (Not printer) (Street, city, county, state, and ZIP+4®)

ELSEVIER INC.
230 Park Avenue, Suite 800
New York, NY 10169

Contact Person
Malathi Samayan

Telephone (Include area code)
91-44-4299-4507

8. Complete Mailing Address of Headquarters or General Business Office of Publisher (Not printer)

ELSEVIER INC.
230 Park Avenue, Suite 800
New York, NY 10169

9. Full Names and Complete Mailing Addresses of Publisher, Editor, and Managing Editor (Do not leave blank)

Publisher (Name and complete mailing address)

Dolores Meloni, ELSEVIER INC.
1600 JOHN F KENNEDY BLVD. SUITE 1600
PHILADELPHIA, PA 19103-2899

Editor (Name and complete mailing address)

Stacy Eastman, ELSEVIER INC.
1600 JOHN F KENNEDY BLVD. SUITE 1600
PHILADELPHIA, PA 19103-2899

Managing Editor (Name and complete mailing address)

PATRICK MANLEY, ELSEVIER INC.
1600 JOHN F KENNEDY BLVD. SUITE 1600
PHILADELPHIA, PA 19103-2899

10. Owner (Do not leave blank. If the publication is owned by a corporation, give the name and address of the corporation immediately followed by the names and addresses of all stockholders owning or holding 1 percent or more of the total amount of stock. If not owned by a corporation, give the names and addresses of the individual owners. If owned by a partnership or other unincorporated firm, give its name and address as well as those of each individual owner. If the publication is published by a nonprofit organization, give its name and address.)

Full Name	Complete Mailing Address
WHOLLY OWNED SUBSIDIARY OF REED/ELSEVIER, US HOLDINGS	1600 JOHN F KENNEDY BLVD. SUITE 1600 PHILADELPHIA, PA 19103-2899

11. Known Bondholders, Mortgagees, and Other Security Holders Owning or Holding 1 Percent or More of Total Amount of Bonds, Mortgages, or Other Securities. If none, check box ▶ ☐ None

Full Name	Complete Mailing Address
N/A	

12. Tax Status (For completion by nonprofit organizations authorized to mail at nonprofit rates) (Check one)
The purpose, function, and nonprofit status of this organization and the exempt status for federal income tax purposes:
☒ Has Not Changed During Preceding 12 Months
☐ Has Changed During Preceding 12 Months (Publisher must submit explanation of change with this statement)

PS Form 3526, July 2014 (Page 1 of 4 (see instructions page 4)) PSN: 7530-01-000-9931   PRIVACY NOTICE: See our privacy policy on www.usps.com.

---

13. Publication Title	14. Issue Date for Circulation Data Below
CLINICS IN PLASTIC SURGERY	AUGUST 2023

15. Extent and Nature of Circulation

			Average No. Copies Each Issue During Preceding 12 Months	No. Copies of Single Issue Published Nearest to Filing Date
a. Total Number of Copies (Net press run)			268	235
b. Paid Circulation (By Mail and Outside the Mail)	(1)	Mailed Outside-County Paid Subscriptions Stated on PS Form 3541 (Include paid distribution above nominal rate, advertiser's proof copies, and exchange copies)	131	116
	(2)	Mailed In-County Paid Subscriptions Stated on PS Form 3541 (Include paid distribution above nominal rate, advertiser's proof copies, and exchange copies)	0	0
	(3)	Paid Distribution Outside the Mails Including Sales Through Dealers and Carriers, Street Vendors, Counter Sales, and Other Paid Distribution Outside USPS®	81	73
	(4)	Paid Distribution by Other Classes of Mail Through the USPS (e.g., First-Class Mail®)	0	0
c. Total Paid Distribution (Sum of 15b (1), (2), (3), and (4)) ▶			214	169
d. Free or Nominal Rate Distribution (By Mail and Outside the Mail)	(1)	Free or Nominal Rate Outside-County Copies Included on PS Form 3541	33	25
	(2)	Free or Nominal Rate In-County Copies Included on PS Form 3541	0	0
	(3)	Free or Nominal Rate Copies Mailed at Other Classes Through the USPS (e.g., First-Class Mail)	0	0
	(4)	Free or Nominal Rate Distribution Outside the Mail (Carriers or other means)	33	25
e. Total Free or Nominal Rate Distribution (Sum of 15d (1), (2), (3) and (4)) ▶			33	25
f. Total Distribution (Sum of 15c and 15e) ▶			247	214
g. Copies not Distributed (See Instructions to Publishers #4 (page #3)) ▶			21	21
h. Total (Sum of 15f and g) ▶			268	235
i. Percent Paid (15c divided by 15f times 100) ▶			86.63%	85.31%

* If you are claiming electronic copies, go to line 16 on page 3. If you are not claiming electronic copies, skip to line 17 on page 3.

16. Electronic Copy Circulation		Average No. Copies Each Issue During Preceding 12 Months	No. Copies of Single Issue Published Nearest to Filing Date
a. Paid Electronic Copies ▶			
b. Total Paid Print Copies (Line 15c) + Paid Electronic Copies (Line 16a) ▶			
c. Total Print Distribution (Line 15f) + Paid Electronic Copies (Line 16a) ▶			
d. Percent Paid (Both Print & Electronic Copies) (16b divided by 16c × 100) ▶			

☒ I certify that 50% of all my distributed copies (electronic and print) are paid above a nominal price.

17. Publication of Statement of Ownership
☒ If the publication is a general publication, publication of this statement is required. Will be printed in the October 2023 issue of this publication.   ☐ Publication not required.

18. Signature and Title of Editor, Publisher, Business Manager, or Owner

Malathi Samayan

Malathi Samayan - Distribution Controller

Date 9/18/2023

I certify that all information furnished on this form is true and complete. I understand that anyone who furnishes false or misleading information on this form or who omits material or information requested on the form may be subject to criminal sanctions (including fines and imprisonment) and/or civil sanctions (including civil penalties).

PS Form 3526, July 2014 (Page 2 of 4)   PRIVACY NOTICE: See our privacy policy on www.usps.com

Moving?

Make sure your subscription moves with you!

To notify us of your new address, find your **Clinics Account Number** (located on your mailing label above your name), and contact customer service at:

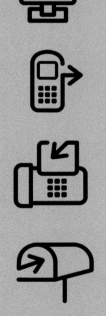

Email: journalscustomerservice-usa@elsevier.com

800-654-2452 (subscribers in the U.S. & Canada)
314-447-8871 (subscribers outside of the U.S. & Canada)

Fax number: 314-447-8029

Elsevier Health Sciences Division
Subscription Customer Service
3251 Riverport Lane
Maryland Heights, MO 63043

*To ensure uninterrupted delivery of your subscription, please notify us at least 4 weeks in advance of move.

9780443130632